THE FEEL GOOD GUIDE

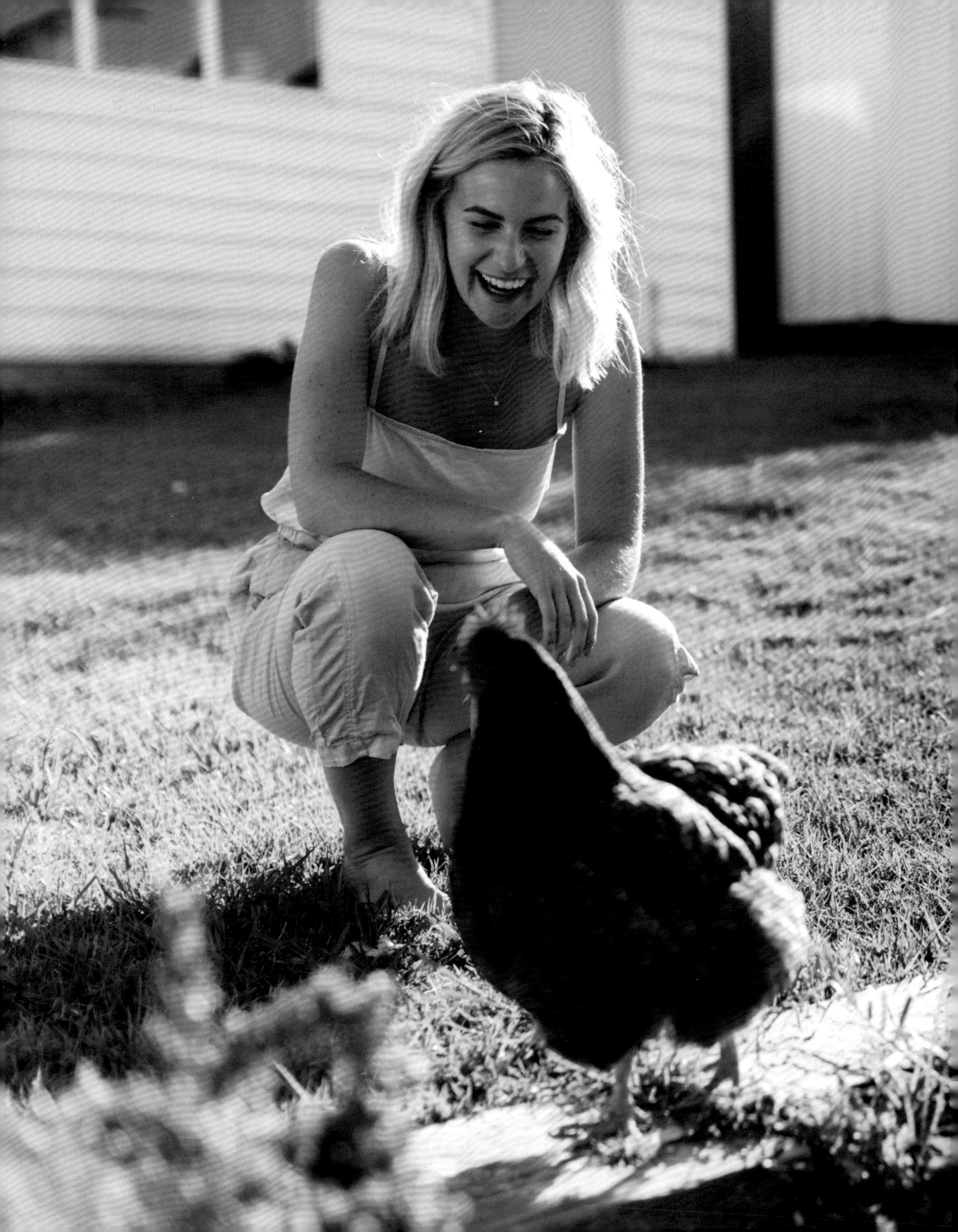

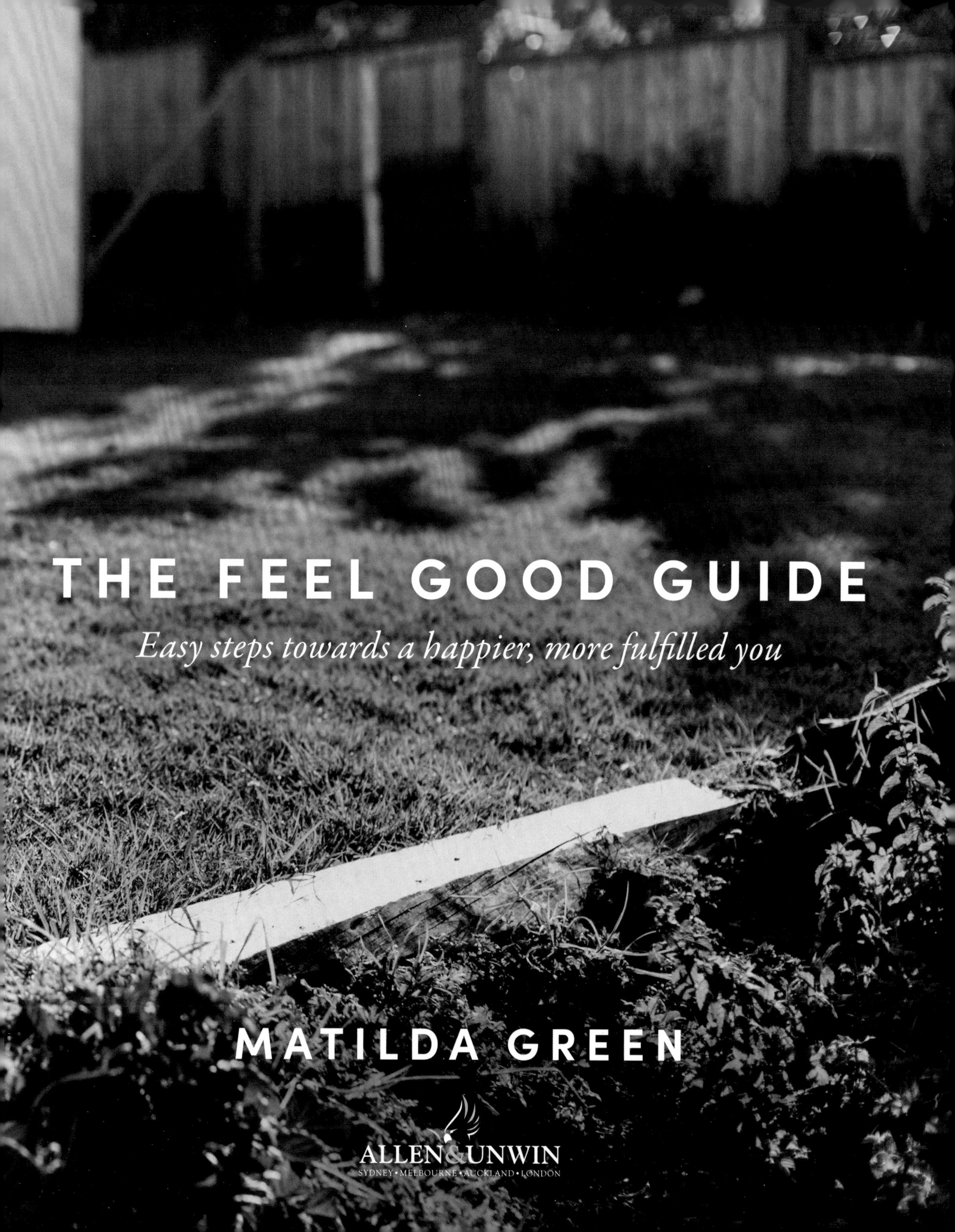

THE FEEL GOOD GUIDE

Easy steps towards a happier, more fulfilled you

MATILDA GREEN

ALLEN&UNWIN
SYDNEY • MELBOURNE • AUCKLAND • LONDON

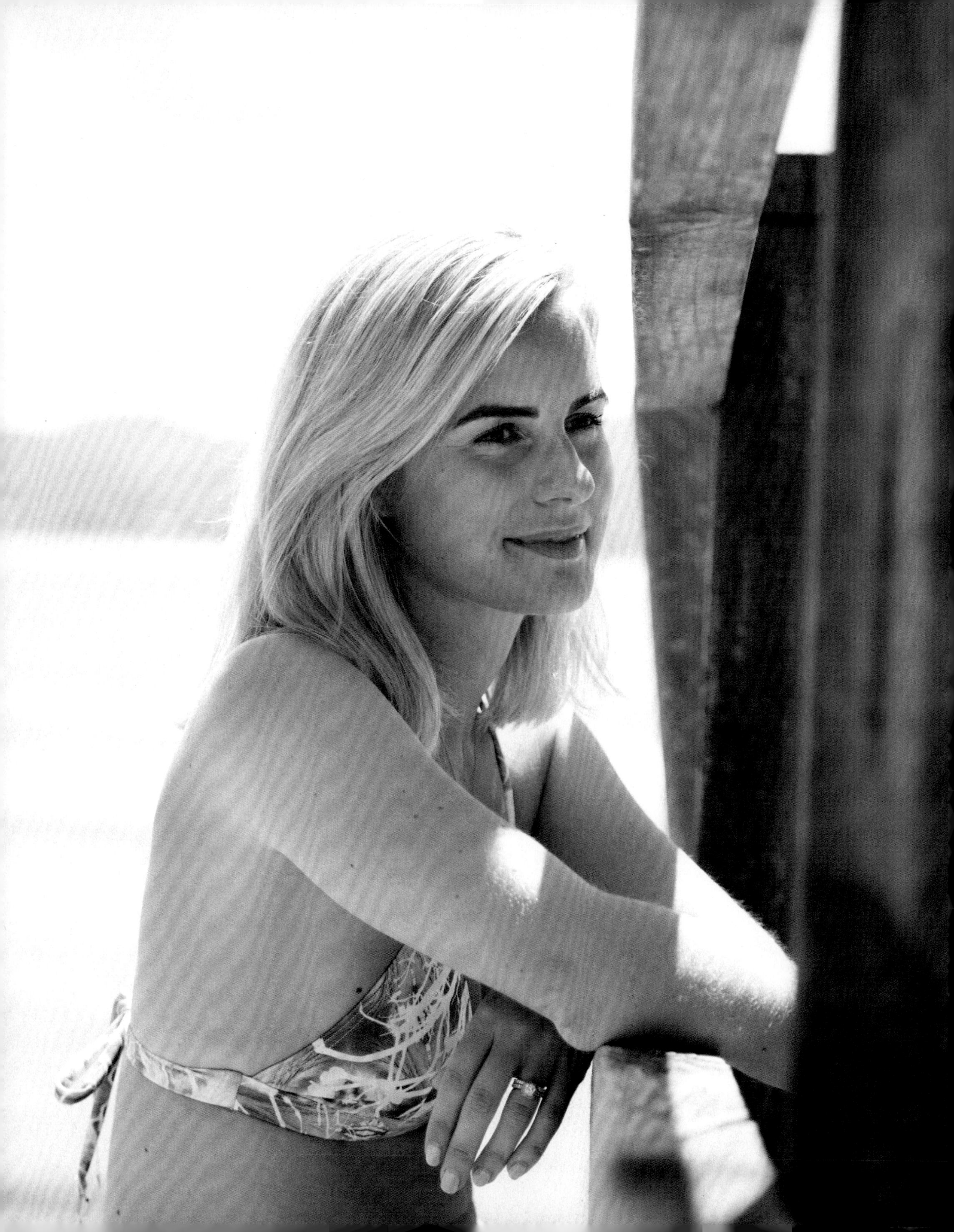

CONTENTS

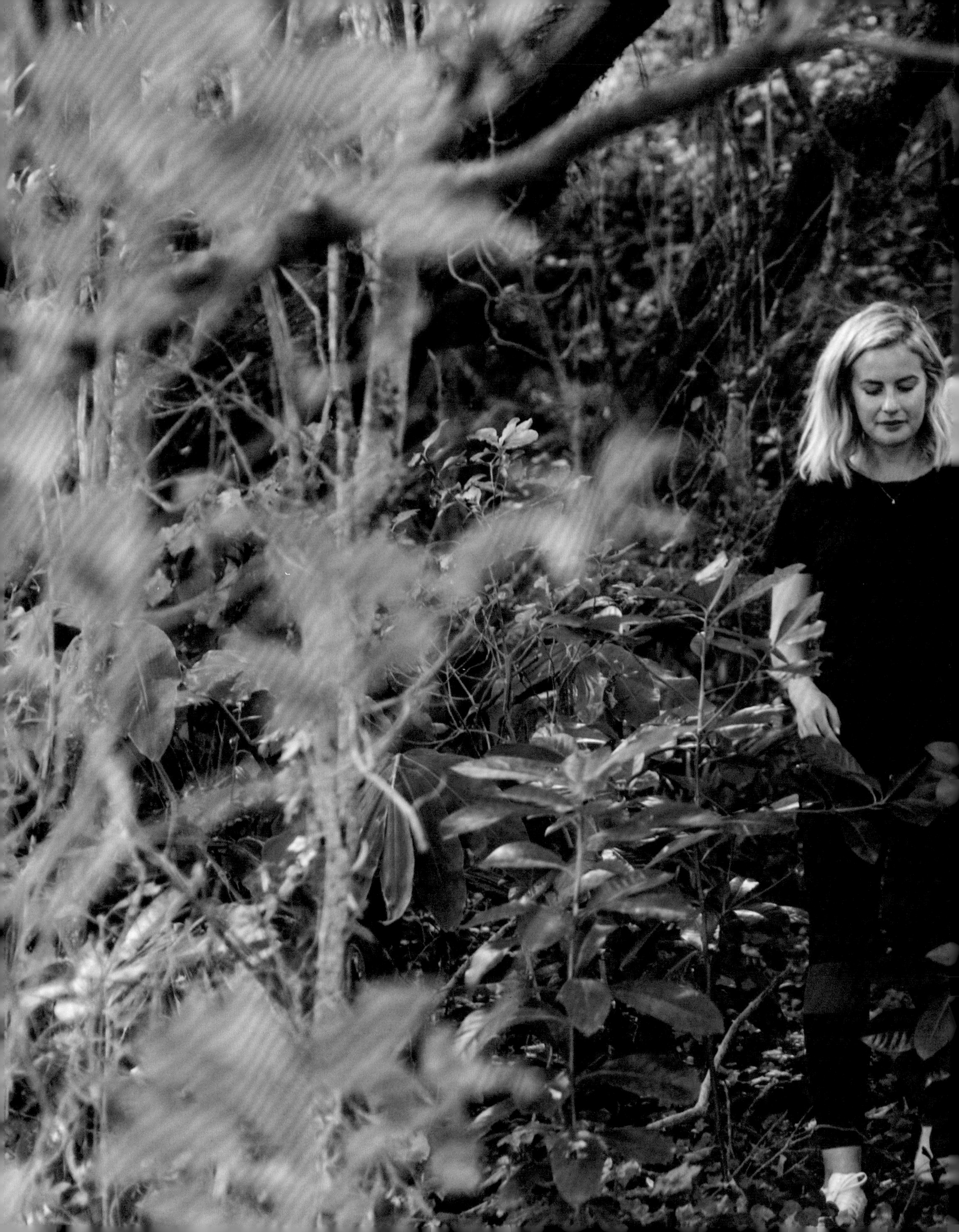

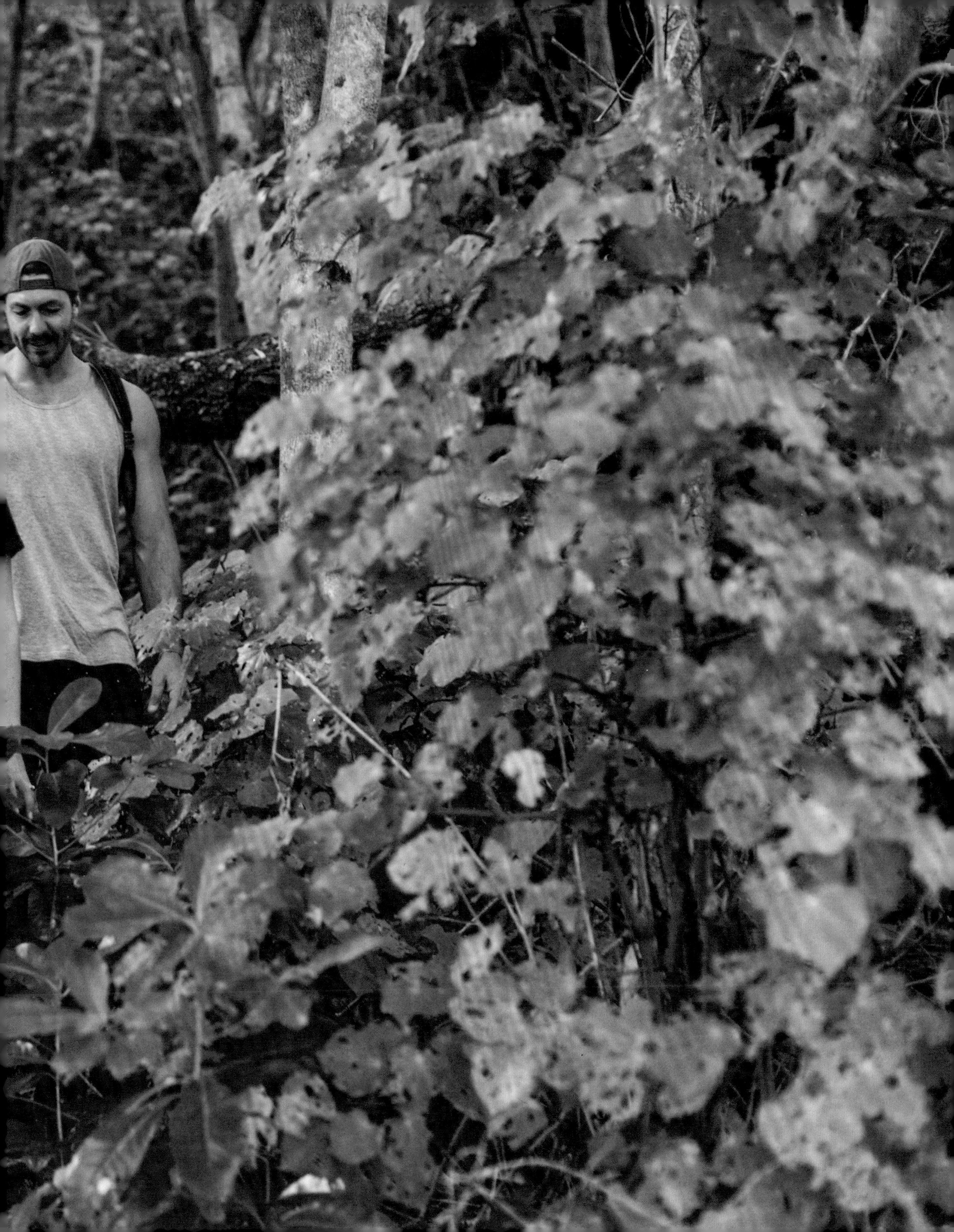

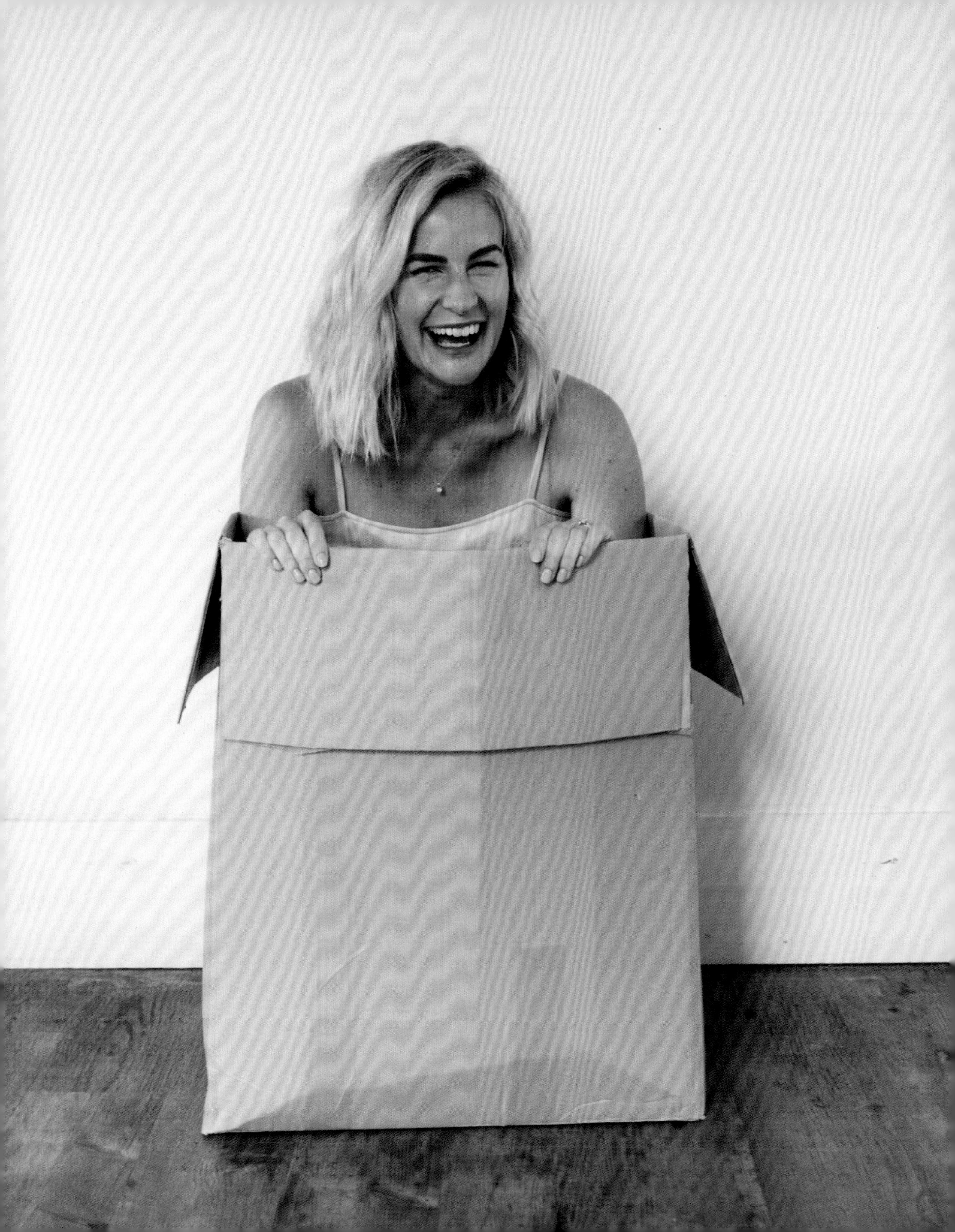

HELLO THERE!

Welcome to *The Feel Good Guide*. Nice to have you here with me!

I've been on a bit of a journey of self-discovery over the last few years, partly as a result of realising that some of the traits that I thought were 'just a part of me' were actually manifestations of weak self-esteem. You know, things like feeling jealous of others, shunning new experiences and adventures, and being incredibly vulnerable to criticism. (More on all this later.)

Chances are that, like me, you've experienced issues with your self-esteem at some stage over your lifetime. We all have. You might even be experiencing them now. If so, you are not alone! As a matter of fact, hordes of us struggle with our self-esteem—even if, from the outside, you'd never guess it. It can be especially hard to believe that other people have self-esteem issues in the digital world we live in, where we're bombarded with other people's seemingly perfect lives all over social media, but the truth is that we all struggle sometimes. In this book, I want to show you how to rise above that drive towards constant comparison, and free yourself from the prison of low self-esteem.

Having strong self-esteem is super important, as it influences so many aspects of your life. It can improve your relationships with your friends and loved ones, it can have a positive impact on your work life, and it can help improve your general happiness.

In this book, I'll share with you some of the things I have learnt on my self-discovery adventure that have helped me to build strong self-esteem. I'm a big believer in learning from the experiences of others, so that's why I've pulled together all of my own experiences here. I hope that, just as they have helped shape my strong self-esteem, they will help you too.

This book isn't about making yourself into a different person. (I wouldn't bloody dream of such a thing.) It's not so much about changing who you are as it is about loving who you are. It's about celebrating your wonderful self, embracing and being proud of the person who you have grown to be, and giving you the tools that help you to remember just how bloody awesome you really are. I hope it'll also help you find ways to make your star shine a bit brighter, if that's what you need.

In each chapter, you'll find an action plan (or two!). These action plans are lists of things that you can start doing tomorrow—or even right now, if you're a keen bean—in order to begin improving your relationship with yourself, and therefore improving your life. I've included these action plans because I truly believe that actions speak louder than words. It's all very well for me to sit here and tell you all of the ways I've built up my own self-esteem, but I think advice needs to come with practical suggestions too. That way, you can read what I have to say, then put the things you want to into action, and start feeling more in control of your own self-esteem and your life in general.

There's a popular saying that the definition of insanity is doing the same thing over and over again, but expecting different results. Don't keep doing the same thing if it's clearly not working. Be open to making the changes you need to if your self-esteem isn't its best. At the end of the day, you can read all the books in the world, but change starts with you.

I believe in you. Now let's make you believe in you.

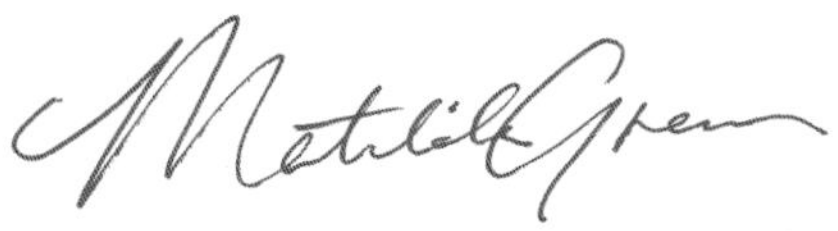

It's about celebrating
your wonderful self,
embracing and being
proud of the person who
you have grown to be.

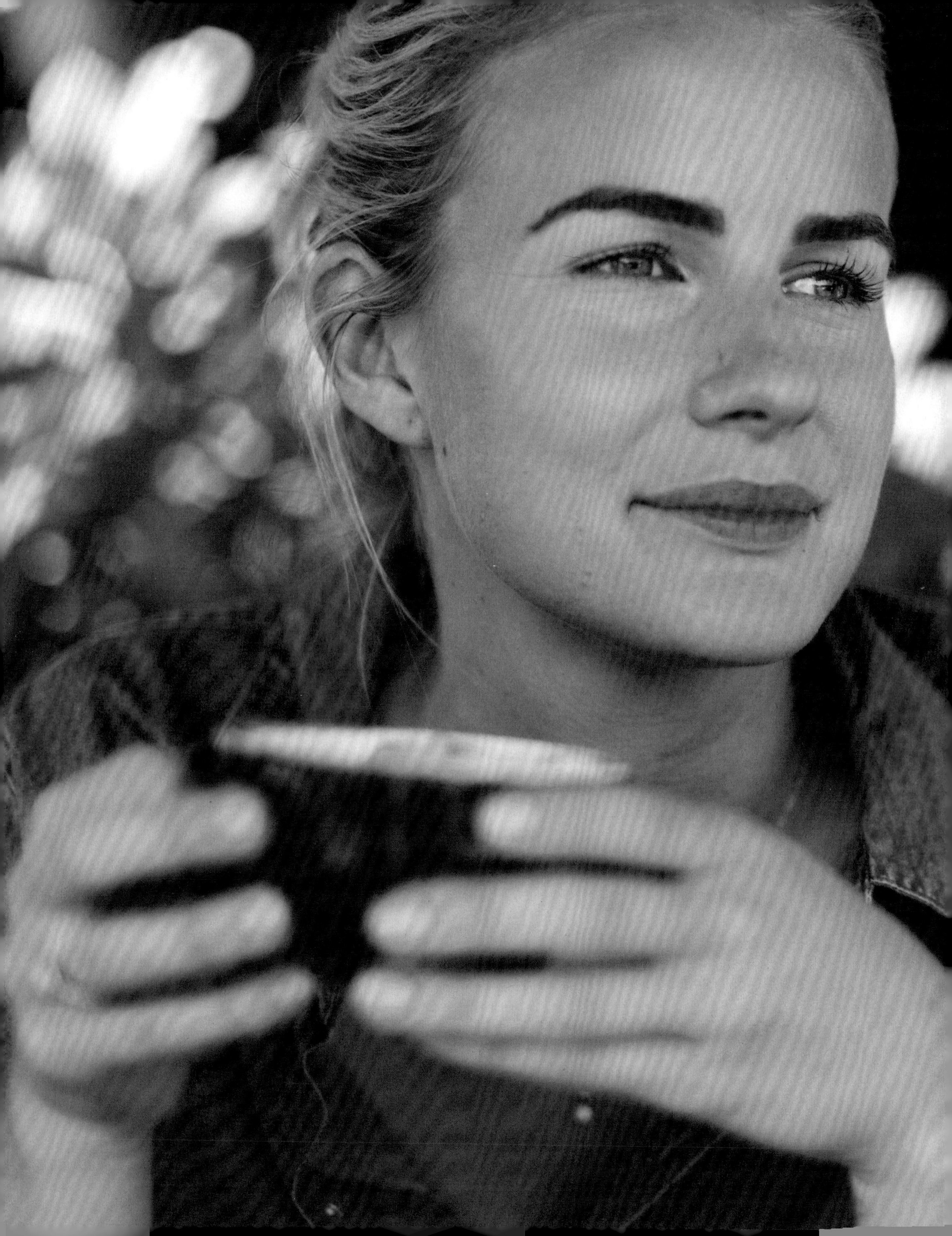

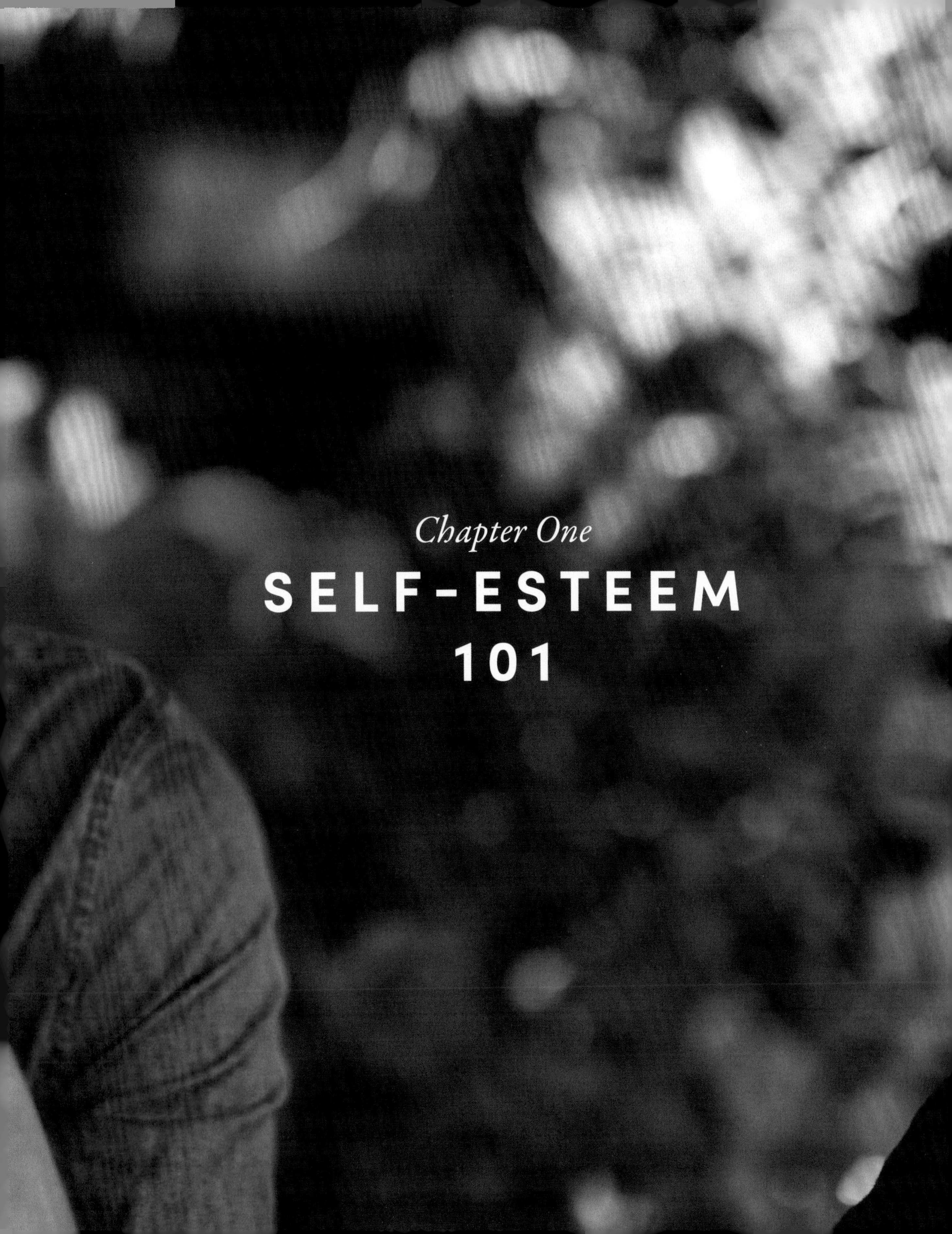

Chapter One

SELF-ESTEEM 101

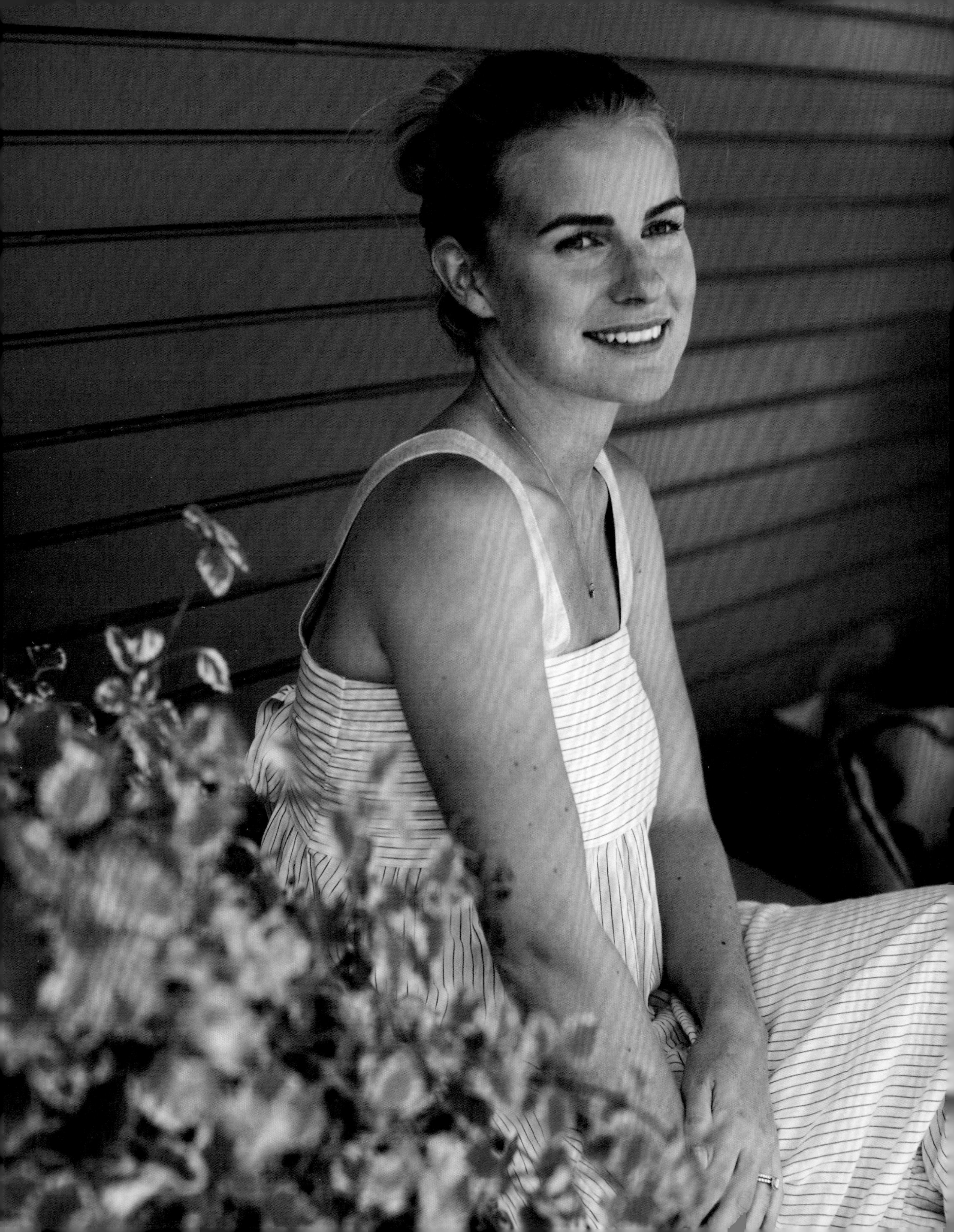

Let's crack right into it, shall we? So, strong self-esteem. What is it? Feeling good about yourself. Loving yourself. Having confidence in your own worth and abilities. Sort of obvious, right? Well, even if it is an easy thing to define, it's not always so easy to actually put into practice.

The fact is that heaps of us battle with our self-esteem, and for all kinds of reasons. That's because a lot of the things that affect self-esteem aren't even related to anything in the outside world, and have everything to do with what's going on in our own little heads. It has nothing to do with whether we have achieved certain goals, or have a certain wardrobe, or have the perfect boyfriend or girlfriend, or whatever it is that we think is going to make us feel happier and better about ourselves.

Self-esteem is kind of like a little voice in your head that tells you things about yourself—and, when your self-esteem is low, it tells you all kinds of nasty stuff that's not true. Let me just repeat that last bit: that's not true. If your self-esteem voice is telling you mean stuff, it's a liar.

These days, a lot of us seem to spend so much of our time wishing that we were different from how we are, that our lives were more interesting, that our bodies were better . . . The list goes on. A lot of the time, these thoughts centre specifically on how we look. We want to change our bodies, we wish we had better clothes, and we start to think that if only we could change certain things about ourselves then our lives would be better. *We* would be better. We hate ourselves if we're not 'perfect', and we compare ourselves to people who we think are perfect. We make promises to lose X amount of weight, or to go to the gym X number of times a week, or to not eat X foods . . . and then, because we are human beings, we break our promises to ourselves and we hate ourselves even more. It's a vicious cycle, people!

Before we go too much further, though, I have an inkling as to what you may be thinking right now. Maybe it's something along the lines of, 'But you're young, blonde, white. What do you have to worry about? What do you know about bad self-esteem?'

You're not the first person to say (or think) something like this. Whenever I've spoken about self-esteem, I've experienced my fair share of comments along these lines and, to be honest, I think they're missing the point. The fact that I am all of these things and *still* have battles with self-esteem just shows how prolific and indiscriminate self-esteem problems really are. Like everyone, I have definitely had my own struggles with self-esteem. It hasn't always been smooth sailing.

Someone might appear to have it all from the outside (cough, social media, cough), but that doesn't tell us anything about what's really going on in their head. It's something to keep in mind the next time you see a post from your pal who looks like they've got everything—it's entirely possible that they've got pretty crappy self-esteem themselves, despite appearances.

THE COMPARISON EFFECT

According to my mum, I was always a very happy child. I didn't cry much, and I laughed a lot—which, of course, was a dream come true for her! But, as I got older and eventually became a teenager, I started to develop an unhealthy habit

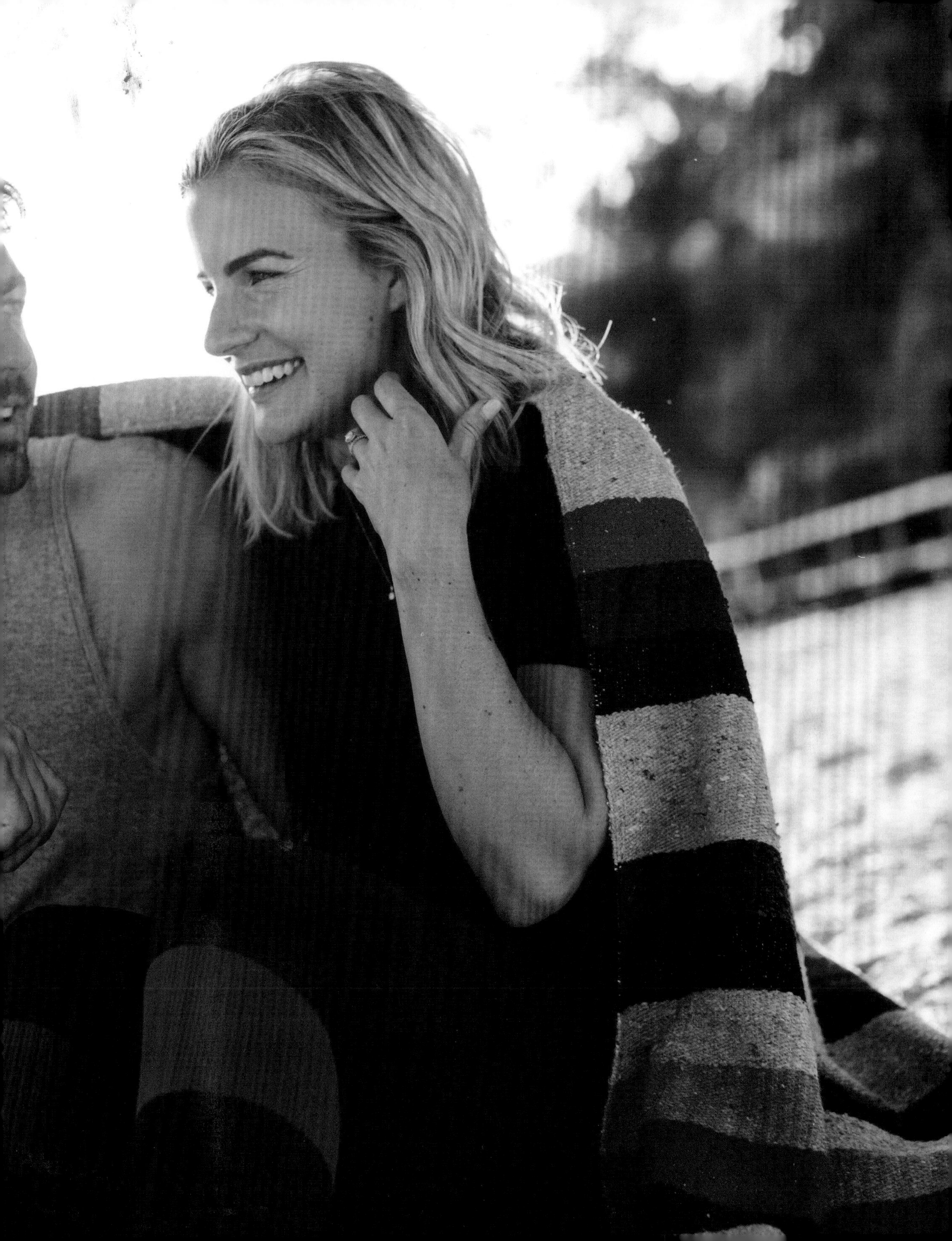

Our uniqueness is the
beautiful foundation of what
it is to be human, and our
differences are what make this
world a really wonderful place.

of comparing myself to others. Not surprisingly, my self-esteem took a bit of a hammering as a result.

There was a lot I didn't like about my appearance when I was in high school. For starters, I was really thin, and I hated it, so I used to wear leggings under my jeans to make my body look curvier. (The irony of this, given the stupid restrictive diets I'd do in later years, is not lost on me.) What's more, I would *never* leave the house without wearing make-up and straightening my hair. All of my friends had straight hair, and I hated my naturally wavy hair. When I look back on those days, it's sort of incredible that everyone was so bloody terrified to stand out in any way whatsoever. I can't help but wonder why that was. Everyone just wanted to be the same as everyone else, because no one realised that we should celebrate our differences.

Our uniqueness is the beautiful foundation of what it is to be human, and our differences are what make this world a really wonderful place. It gets said all the time, but imagine how boring things would be if we were all the same. No, really—take a moment to stop and imagine it. Imagine if we all had the same colour hair, the same type of skin, the same beliefs, the same preferences and likes and dislikes. There would be no excitement!

If you ever find yourself comparing your life, your body, your whatever to other people's, remember this little gem: it's the things that are different about you that make you the person you are. And, for that reason, it's important to embrace the things about you that make you different from your family, your friends, the people you follow on social media. Celebrate those differences. (The same goes on the flip side: embrace the differences of those around you. Celebrate them. Encourage other people to be themselves.)

Anyway, back to comparison and my high-school days . . . I was fortunate enough to go to a private high school, but that also meant I was surrounded by some incredibly wealthy families. I'd often compare myself to the wealthier kids and think, *I wish I had as much as them*. I felt a bit average, because I thought I didn't measure up and my clothes weren't expensive enough.

I know exactly what you're thinking. A private-school girl wishing she was better off? I can almost hear your eyes rolling in to the back of your head, and I completely agree—it's ludicrous. But it's also the perfect example of how ridiculous this temptation to compare yourself to others really is. It's also a reminder that every experience is relative to the person going through it. Even when you've got things pretty good, you can still find yourself wishing you had more, or that things were different.

If you get stuck in a rut of comparing yourself to other people, you're always going to find ways that you or your life don't seem to measure up—no matter how many good things are already around you. You know that saying that there are always people better and worse off than you? Well, that one evaporates into thin air the moment we start comparing ourselves to other people. Everyone suddenly *seems* more accomplished and better looking, *seems* to have a better job and a nicer house, *seems* more physically fit or to have more money, or just *seems* to be generally happier in their lives. The key word there is 'seems'. It's not the real thing, now, is it?

I like to call this the 'comparison effect'. It's what happens when you compare yourself to other people who seem to have more than you, without knowing anything about their personal lives. All it does is make you feel bad about yourself.

Of course, because our whole world has been taken over by social media platforms like Instagram and Facebook, it can be hard to avoid seeing how perfect other people's lives are (or, at least, how perfect they seem!). The comparison effect might have started in high school for me, but it really ramped up when social media became a big part of my life and work. Now, we're so inundated with everyone's best angles, their lush holidays (unsure if people still say lush any more?) and their happy moments that it becomes increasingly easy to forget that EVERYONE has problems. Common sense tells us that nobody's life is perfect, but for some reason that seems to go out the window as soon as we start scrolling through our social media feeds.

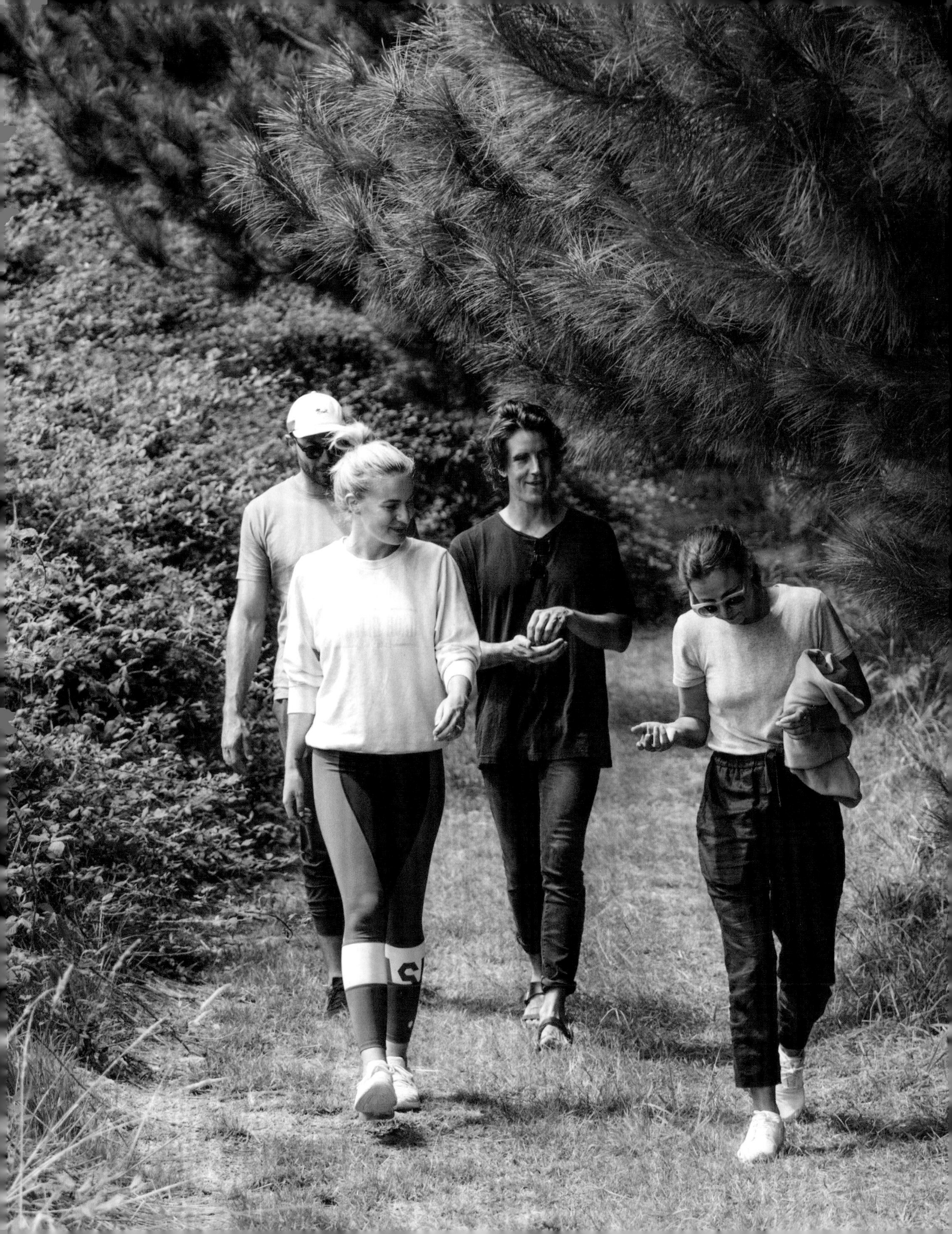

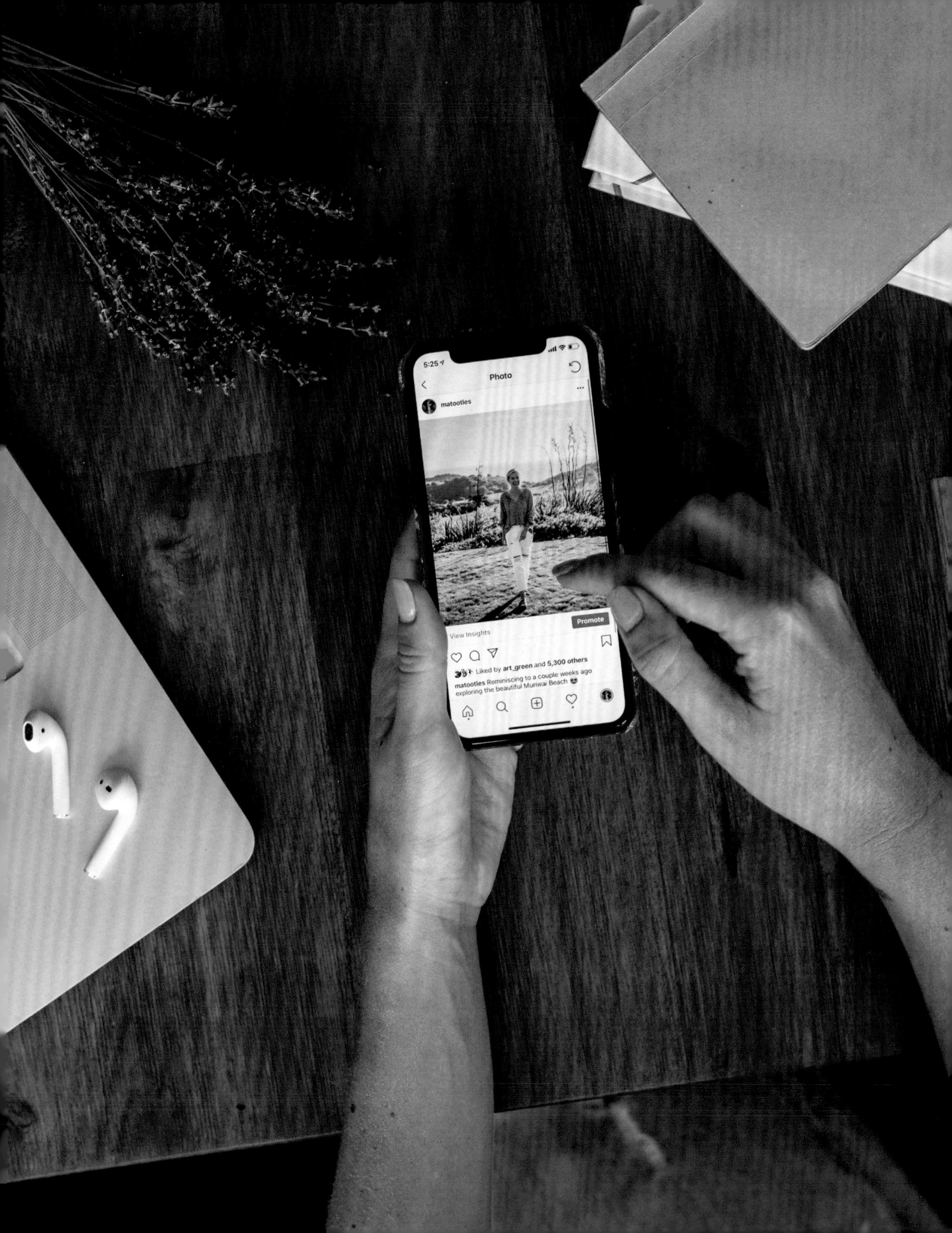
5:25
Photo
matootles
Promote
View Insights
Liked by art_green and 5,300 others
matootles Reminiscing to a couple weeks ago exploring the beautiful Muriwai Beach

SOCIAL MEDIA VS SELF-ESTEEM

When it comes to social media, lots of us only share the nice stuff from our lives. We don't always want to post the sad stuff—but that can mean that our feeds just end up looking like everything's sunshine and happiness all the time. Of course, ain't nothing wrong with sunshine and happiness . . . until you start looking at the feeds of the people you follow, think that's all there is in their lives, and then feel bad because your life isn't as good, or wonder why they don't seem to have bad days like you do. That sneaky little voice creeps into your head and tells you it's because something's wrong with you, and your self-esteem plummets. We've all been there.

I'm sure there are people out there who would just say, 'Well, if social media makes you feel so bad about yourself, why not just quit it then?' To which I'd reply by stating the obvious: quitting social media is just not that easy for many of us. For lots of us (ahem, me) social media is a massive part of our jobs. And, even if it's not, chances are it's one of the main ways you stay in touch with people, and keep up to date with what your friends and family are doing. Dropping out of social media might work for some people, but it can also come at a cost—and not all of us are willing to pay that price.

To give you an idea of just how much a part of our lives social media has become, let's take a quick look at some numbers. First up, reports released in 2018 by We Are Social and Hootsuite found that:

*   the number of social media users worldwide in 2018 was 3.196 billion. (The total world population is currently 7.7 billion, to put that in perspective.)

*   the average Kiwi spends 5 hours 59 minutes a day on the internet (on any device), and of that they spend 1 hour 53 minutes on social media.

* more than two-thirds of the world's population now has a mobile phone, with most people now using a smartphone.

And then, in terms of how much more common social media has become, earlier this year Pew Research Center released data on social media usage in the US that showed that 65 per cent of adults now use social networking sites— and that's a nearly tenfold jump in the past decade. So, love it or hate it, social media is a big part of the world we live in. You can stop using it, if that's your jam, but you'll be in the minority.

There's a whole lot of chat out there about the impact that social media has on our lives and on our mental health. So, what does science have to say about that? Well, it's a bit of a mixed bag. Social media is still pretty new, so there's not a lot of conclusive data, but what the research does seem to point to is that social media can be both bad for us and good for us. Helpful, huh? It all seems to depend on several factors, including how you use social media, what type of personality you have, and your existing mental health.

Notably, though, there are quite a few studies that suggest that using social media can exacerbate feelings of loneliness—and loneliness definitely isn't good for you. In January 2019, *Forbes* reported on a new study from the University of Pittsburgh and West Virginia University that found that negative experiences on social media were linked to increased feelings of social isolation—or, in other words, when people had bad experiences on social media they felt lonelier. By contrast, the study found that positive experiences had little or no impact. The study's authors suggested this was because of 'negativity bias', or our tendency to remember and be affected by negative events much more strongly than positive ones. The fact we tend to let negative comments or experiences get to us more than positive ones is, in my eyes, a bit of a flaw in human nature. It's a mindset I try to change in myself when I can, but it is really bloody hard. It's like we're hardwired to take criticism or negativity more seriously.

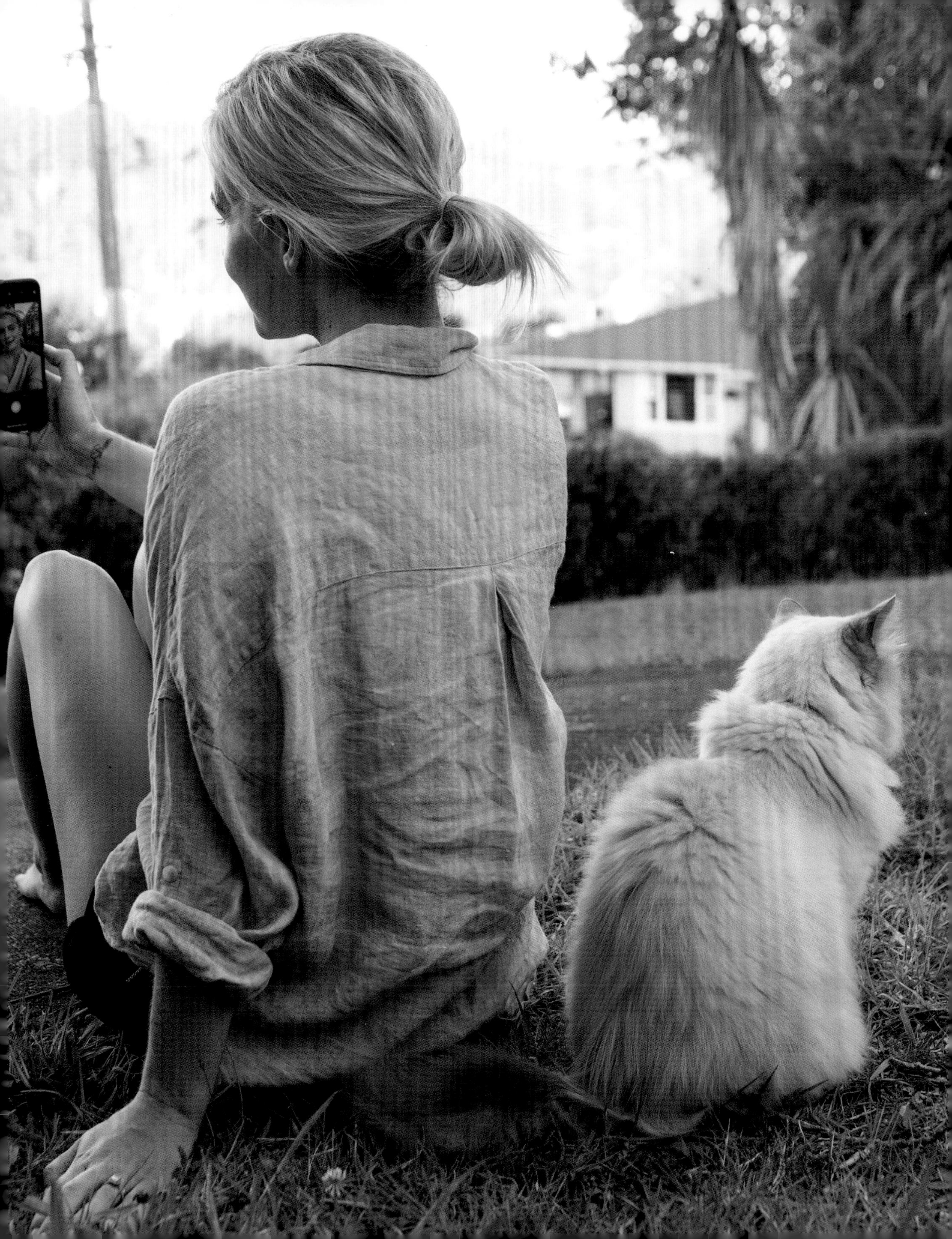

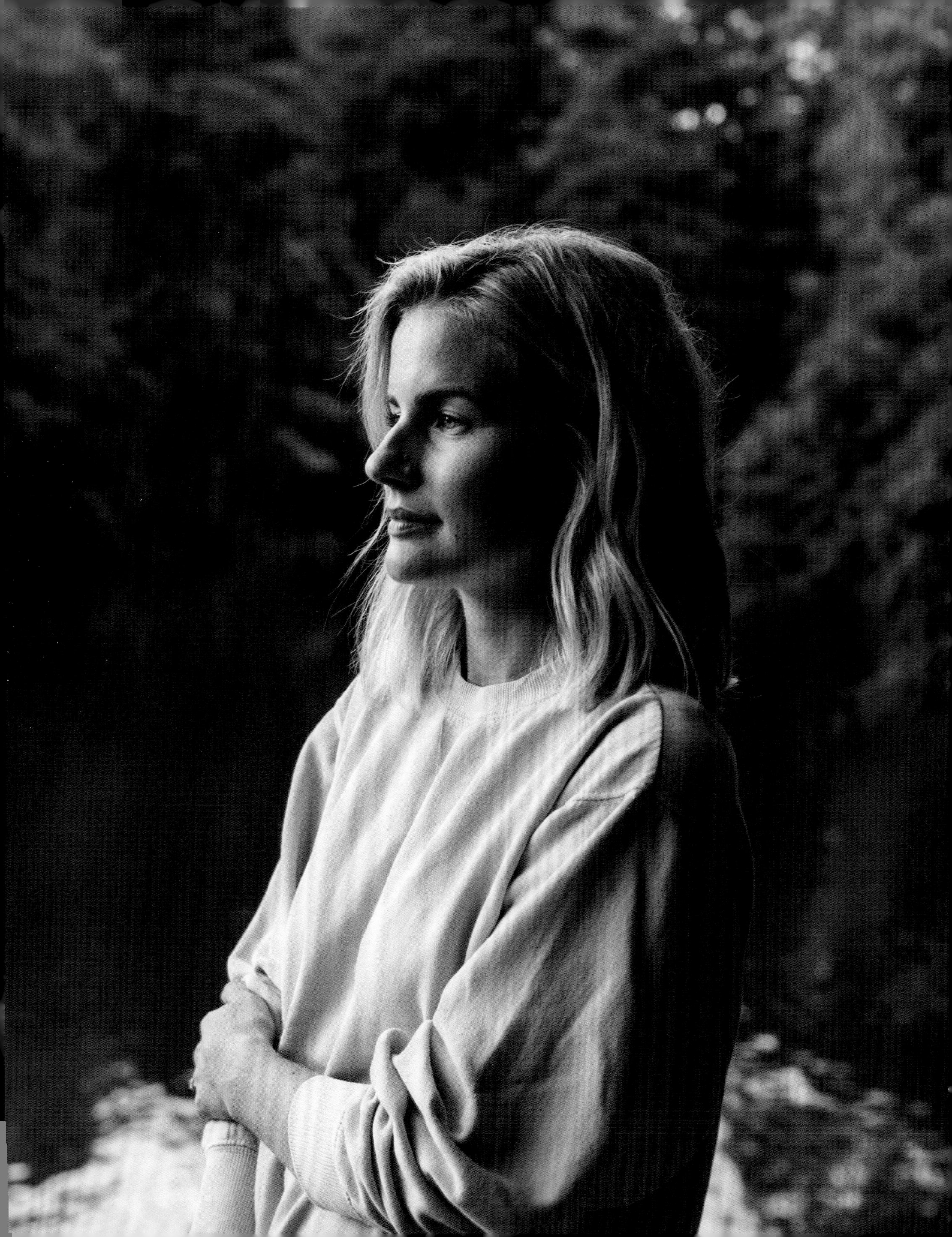

Another study, published in the *American Journal of Preventive Medicine* in 2018, surveyed 7000 19- to 32-year-olds and found that those who spent the most time on social media were twice as likely to report experiencing social isolation. The researchers said that seeing 'such highly idealised representations of peers' lives may cause feelings of envy and the distorted belief that others lead happier and more successful lives, which may increase perceived social isolation.'

In other words, social media can really ramp up the comparison effect by causing you to compare your life to what you think the lives of the people you follow are like, based on their social media feeds. And, sadly, all too often you just feel lonelier and worse about yourself as a result.

There's also research out there that has looked into the impact of social media on things like sleep, our relationships and addiction, and I have to say the verdict's not looking great on any of those fronts. (Although, to be fair, the problem doesn't seem to be just social media on its own—it's also how much time you spend staring at your phone.)

And, just to keep things balanced, there's actually an emerging body of research looking into how social media might be a force for good, for example when it comes to treating things like depression. On this note, I'm sure heaps of you will agree that there is a lot that can be great about social media. It's not all doom and gloom! For example, social media can connect us to lots of incredible people and places that we would possibly have no idea about otherwise. What's more, it also gives creatives, activists and people who run their own businesses a platform to talk to their followers, it entertains and amuses us, and it can put us in touch with communities of like-minded folk we might never have met.

Personally, I've found that social media can also be a source of beautiful empathy and encouragement. Whenever I have posted about feeling low or about going through something difficult, the amount of messages I receive from people offering words of support and love (these are people who I have never even met, might I add) is incredible. These messages far outweigh in number any of the negative messages I have ever received. This always gives me warm fuzzies. I guess that, sometimes, it's just easier for us to speak to a phone than to a real person. We might feel a little more comfortable speaking about how we're feeling when there isn't a real-life human sitting there in front of us, and I think that has opened the door to a really lovely, caring side of social media—which just tells me something about how many lovely, caring humans there are behind all those phones.

SELF-ESTEEM IN THE SPOTLIGHT

I'd started to gain a public profile after appearing on the first season of *The Bachelor New Zealand* back in 2015 when the comparison effect really took hold of me. All of a sudden, all of these people were watching me, following me on Instagram, and I felt as though my life wasn't exciting or glamorous enough to warrant the attention. In order to 'justify' my followers' interest in me, I felt this pressure to live up to a version of myself that was what I thought everyone wanted me to be.

It was a really difficult time. For one, I was dealing with the anxiety I felt as a result of suddenly being in the media and having to live in the public eye. (A New Zealand version of the public eye, of course—it's not as if paparazzi wait outside my house. If they did, I'd imagine they'd pretty quickly get sick of taking photos of me in my trackpants.) At the same time, I was also trying to make my relationship work while it felt like the whole country was judging my every move. I know, I know. This all sounds very dramatic given that New Zealand is a tiny place and 'celebrities' here only have to deal with a fraction of the media attention that international stars do. Even so, I found it really difficult. It was especially hard to deal with getting so many nasty, judgy comments from people on the internet who had never met me

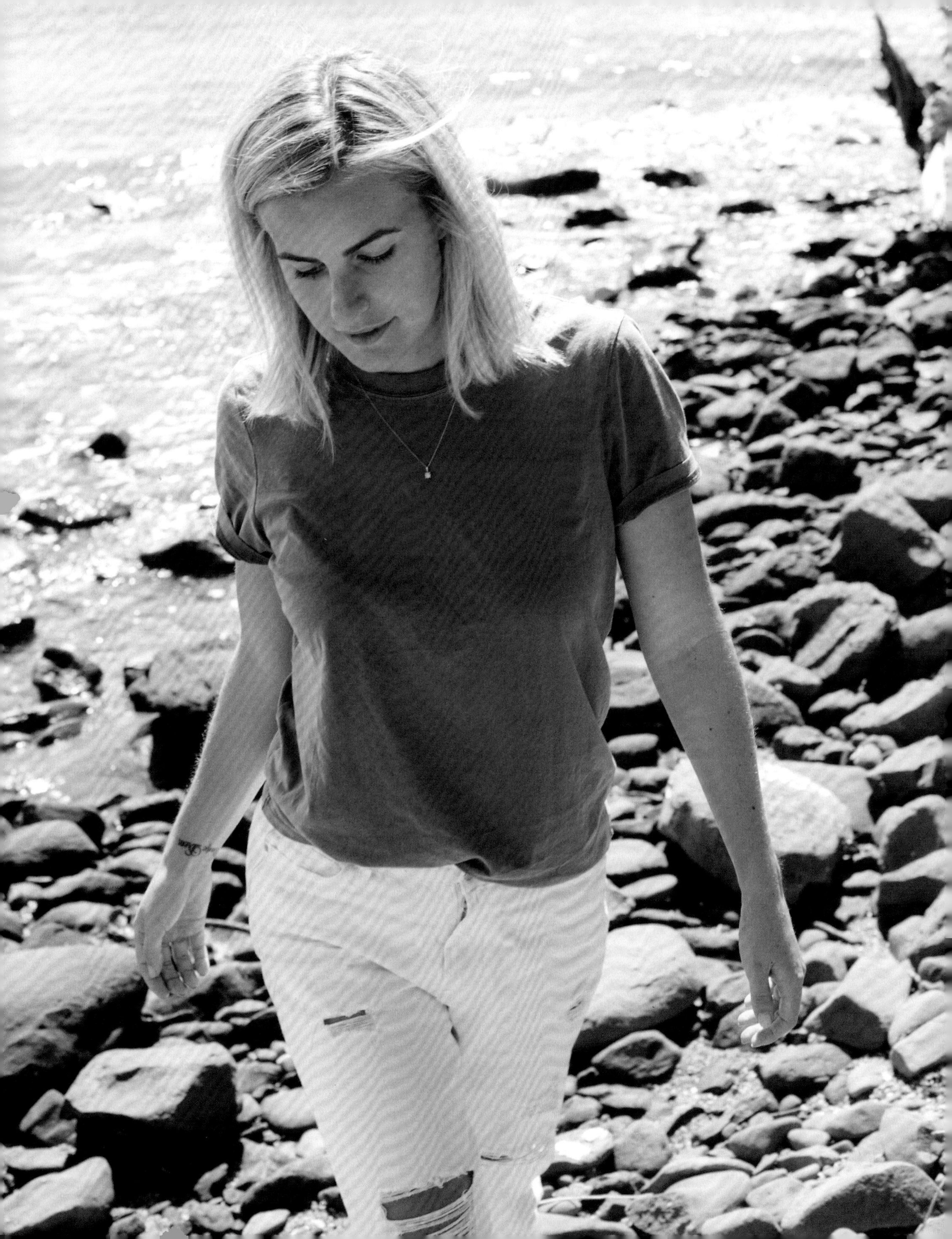

It's taken me a long time to get my self-esteem to the point where I really believe in myself. It's something I've had to work hard on over the years.

(comments that I always insisted on reading—I'm unsure why).

When I look back now, from a much better place in my life, I'm able to see that my anxiety came in part from a deep-seated belief that I wasn't good enough. Have you heard of imposter syndrome? Back then, I didn't have any idea what it was, but when someone mentioned it to me a while ago I immediately looked it up. As I read about it, I found myself nodding along, thinking, *Yup, so me.*

If you haven't heard of it, imposter syndrome is basically when a person doubts their accomplishments or their abilities, and is constantly afraid that they'll suddenly be exposed as a—yep, you guessed it—imposter. There might be a heap of evidence that shows how competent they are, but those who experience imposter syndrome will remain utterly convinced that they are frauds and don't deserve the things they've achieved. They tend to believe that their successes are the result of dumb luck or that they've somehow managed to trick others into thinking they're smarter than they really are. What's more, like poor self-esteem, imposter syndrome doesn't really care who you are. It can get to anyone, and has been shown to affect both men and women.

When I first learnt all this, it made me wonder how many of us are wandering around out there thinking we aren't good enough to be where we are? I even noticed a bit of this sort of thing creeping into my head when I was writing this book—thoughts along the lines of *Why would people want to listen to you, Matilda?* Thankfully, by now I've discovered that one trick when these imposter-ish thoughts creep in is to see them for what they are, and quash them straight away. You just have to drown out that imposter voice with a louder voice. Your voice. A positive, confident voice that says, 'You know what? Why *wouldn't* people listen to me? I have something to say, and by golly I am going to say it. And, if people don't want to listen, then they don't have to.' (You don't have to say 'by golly', but you get the gist.)

It's taken me a long time to get my self-esteem to the point where I really believe in myself. It's something I've had to work hard on over the years, but it's paid off because things have improved significantly. I'm still not a hundred per cent there in terms of never having any self-doubt whatsoever (I'm not sure anyone is, actually), but I'm on the journey. And that's what counts.

IT'S ABOUT THE JOURNEY

As I've mentioned, your self-esteem and your happiness are closely linked. Just like self-esteem, happiness doesn't really have anything to do with material things. You can have a lot of 'things', after all, but still be very unhappy.

Too often, people are busy working towards something they think will make them happy, but happiness isn't a goal. For example, a young woman—let's call her Roberta, shall we?—thinks that if she just keeps slogging away at her shitty job, she'll get promoted, and then she'll make more money, and then she'll be happy. Or maybe Roberta just wants to live in a nicer house, and then she'll be happy. Or maybe Roberta is single and thinks that when she finds a partner, then she'll be happy. This kind of thinking does my head in! I just want to grab Roberta and shake her (gently, of course, but firmly) and yell, 'ROBERTA! YOU'RE MISSING OUT ON LIFE!'

Don't be Roberta. (Unless your name actually is Roberta. In that case, feel free to keep being Roberta, but maybe learn from this book-version of Roberta.) Life is too short to wait for happiness to come to you. It's not a magical destination you will one day reach when you have lots of whatever you think it is you need in order to be happy. Here's the not-so-secret secret: happiness—just like self-esteem—lies in the journey.

If you're searching for happiness on the outside, it's time to stop. I hate to break it to you, but you're not going to find it there. Happiness is something that comes from within, and that's precisely why it's so closely connected to how you feel about yourself. It's been said before, but happiness really is a state of mind. It's also about more than just putting a smile on your face or

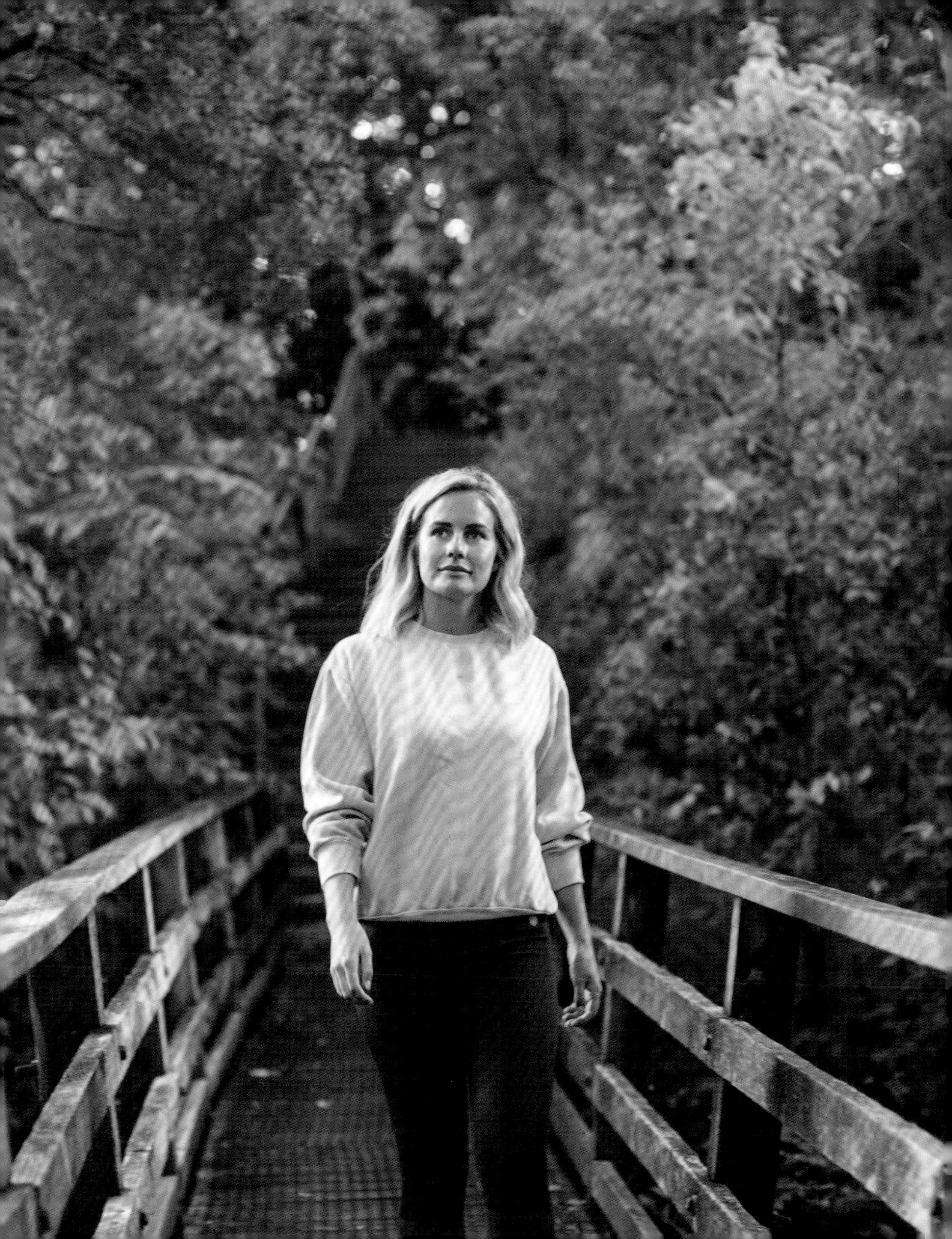

everything going smoothly all the time. Just like good self-esteem, happiness is something you have to work on.

You can't get away with quick fixes here. Going shopping for new clothes might make you ecstatically happy in the short term, but I bet it's only a couple of weeks before that happiness evaporates and you're already sick of those new clothes—and probably just want more. Sound familiar? That is *not* the kind of happiness we're after here. We'll take the long-term contentment instead, thanks!

True happiness isn't about everything being right—or even positive—all the time. It's about learning to be happy and content within ourselves, even when the world might be telling us otherwise. It's about learning to find happiness in the smallest of places, so that we can enjoy the peaks and ride out the troughs of life. Sometimes, it's even about finding happiness at the same time as letting ourselves be sad, or angry, or hurt.

Likewise, strong self-esteem doesn't make you bulletproof. Even after you put heaps of effort into feeling good about yourself, you're still going to have days when you just don't feel the love. And that's fine. It's because you're human. The thing you need is a toolkit of tips and tricks that you can put into action whenever you do feel your self-esteem wavering, so that you can get right back to being your awesome self.

If only such a toolkit of helpful action plans existed . . . Perhaps in the form of a book? You know, sort of like this book?

You, my friend, are in luck. Read on!

True happiness isn't about
everything being right—or
even positive—all the time.
It's about learning to be happy
and content within ourselves,
even when the world might
be telling us otherwise.

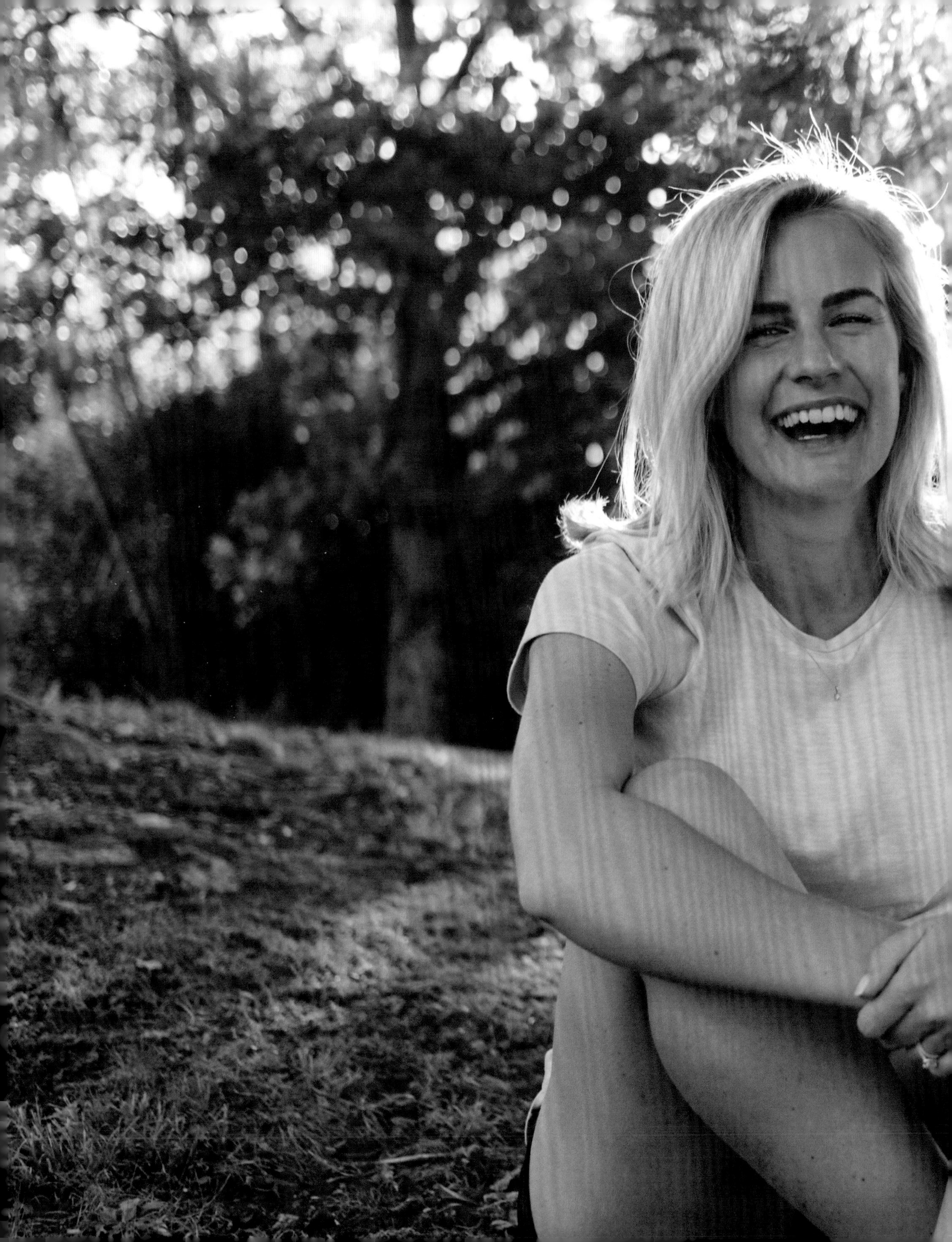

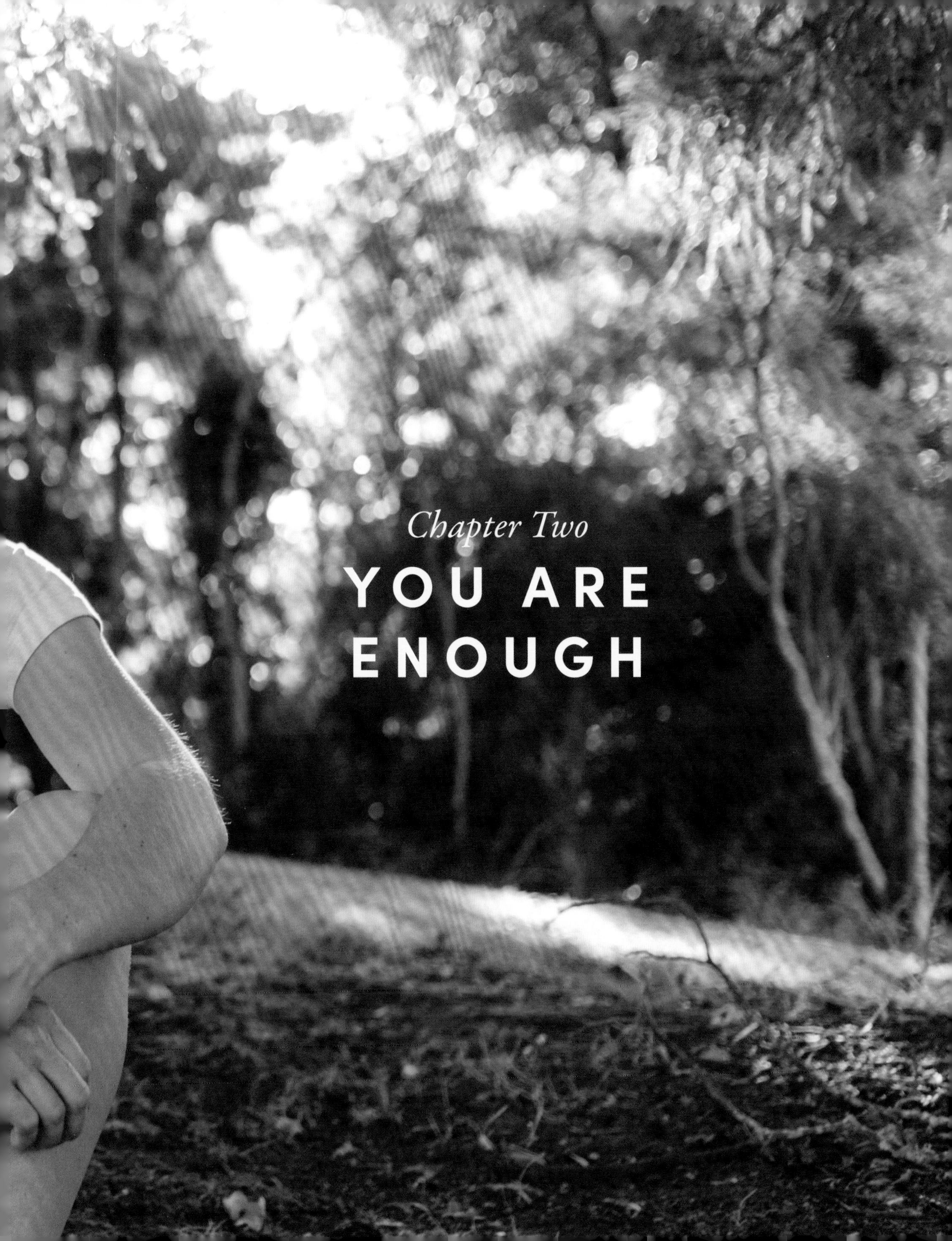

Chapter Two

YOU ARE ENOUGH

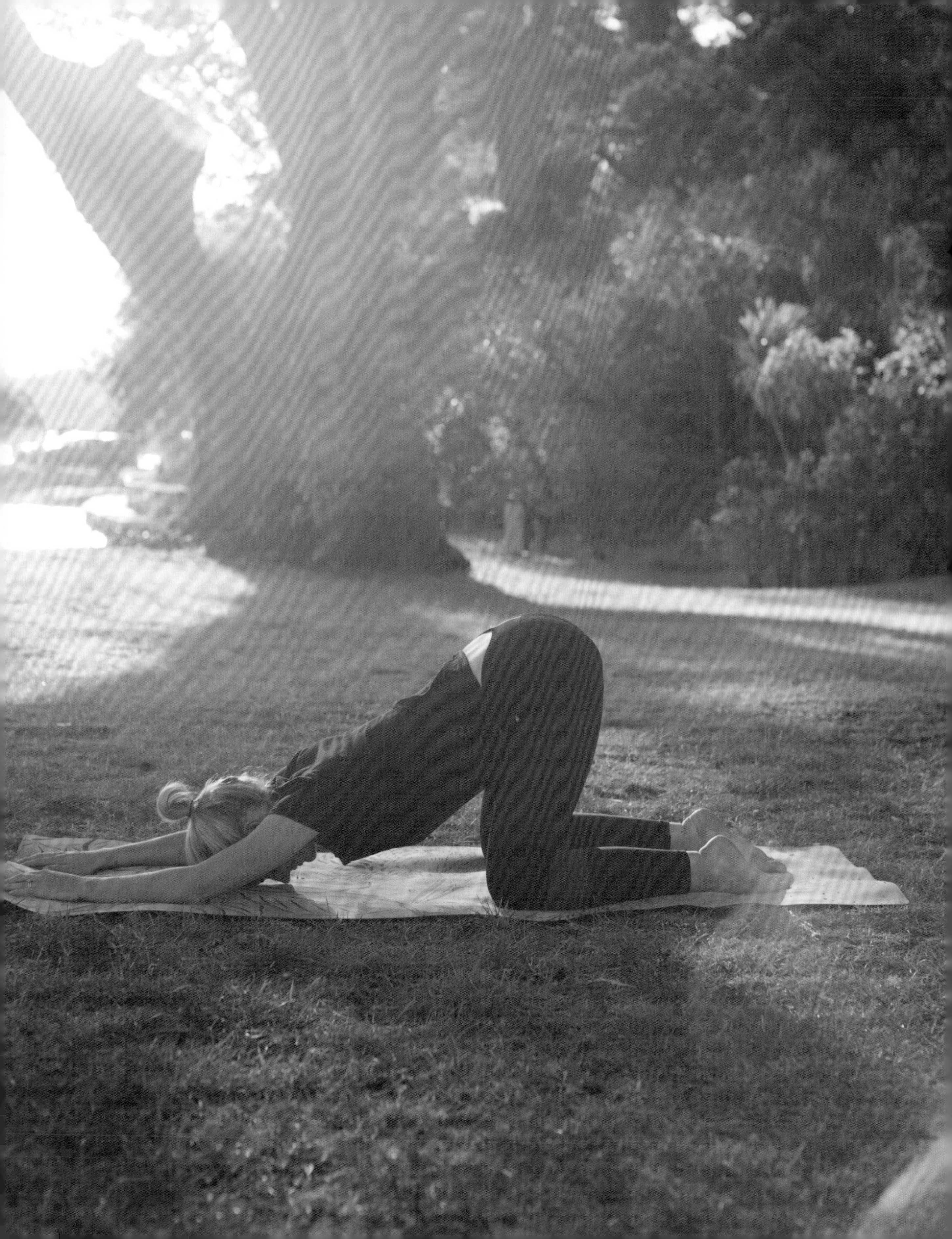

Before you read on, and before I bombard you with action plans for boosting that self-esteem of yours, I want to start with one incredibly important sentiment. This is something that you must never forget: you are enough just as you are. You're already awesome, loved and wonderful. All this book is here to do is remind you of that, and to make you actually *believe* that statement if you don't already.

Sometimes it can take a while to find your self-belief. A lot of the time, it's hidden way deep down inside, and has been pushed down there over the years by negative thoughts and mind-chatter, and by outside forces that encourage you to think you'll never be good enough if you don't look or act a certain way. If this sounds familiar, you simply need to reach down, grab your self-belief with both hands and yank it up above the noise.

It's no good trying to build solid self-esteem if you've got shifty foundations. Remember the three little pigs? It was the third little piggie who finally fended off the wolf because she built her house out of bricks (yes, she's a she in my version). She took the time to do the job properly, even if it took a bit longer, and her hard work paid off. Your self-esteem isn't really all that different from one of those piggies' houses. (Don't worry, these piggies are here to make a point—stay with me!) Do you want self-esteem that will topple at the merest puff of breath from a bloody wolf, or do you want strong and resilient self-esteem that'll stand up to a hurricane?

I'm going to go ahead and assume you'll take the strong one. In that case, be like that smart pig. Take the time to do the job properly, right from the start. And what's the thing that makes a house strong, right from the beginning? The foundations! It's no good loading up all those bricks—or, in the case of your self-esteem, trying to do all the action plans in this book—if there's no base to hold them in place. When it comes to building your self-esteem, there are two very important things you need to lay down before you start trying to do anything else: self-love and self-care.

LOVE YOURSELF

The term self-love is thrown around so much these days, but a lot of people don't really know what it is. Worse, they might have written it off as being just for hippies (and, let me add, there's nothing wrong with being an earth child). Self-love is actually pretty simple. It's just compassion. It's about showing yourself compassion, recognising you're doing your best, and cutting yourself some slack.

How many times have you had friends come to you saying they're stressed, or that they need help, or that they feel overwhelmed? What sort of advice do you give them? I bet it's usually along the lines of, 'Take it easy. Give yourself a break. Remember that you're doing your best.'

Now, here's another question for you: how often do you actually follow your own advice?

A lot of us try too hard to be everything to everyone all the time. But that's not possible for anyone, so something has to take the hit—and that something is usually ourselves. We tend to just put our blinkers on so we can do what needs to be done, and that usually means putting ourselves last (something that's

When it comes to building your self-esteem, there are two very important things you need to lay down before you start trying to do anything else: self-love and self-care.

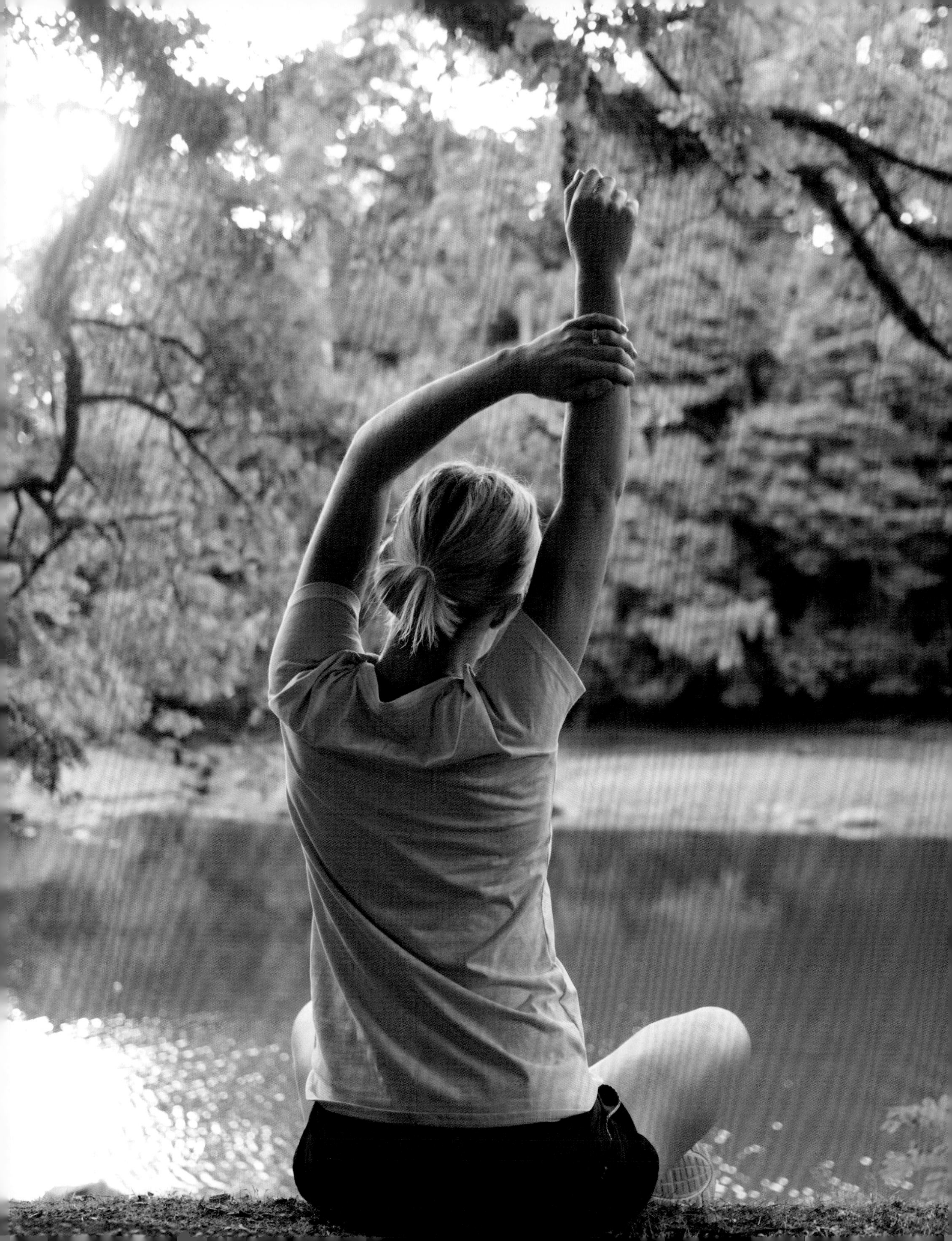

especially relevant to all you parents out there). We are so focused on making sure that everyone else is OK that we can completely forget about making sure that *we* are OK.

If this sounds familiar, welcome to the club! It's time for you to take some time for yourself. Just like everyone else, you are part of this beautiful thing called life and you are trying your best—and sometimes you just need to stop and appreciate that. Appreciate who you are.

Self-love feeds directly (and pretty obviously) into self-esteem. When you look after yourself and love yourself, you build your self-esteem. At the same time, your inner strength and resilience grow, and you become far better equipped to deal with all the things life throws at you. Resilience is definitely a quality that's worth investing some time in: it's what helps you to get back up and carry on whenever life knocks you down. It can seem like resilience is something that you either have or you don't, but that's not really true. Like self-esteem, resilience is something that you can grow. And do you wanna know what some of the factors are that psychologists (in other words, the pros) say make a person resilient? A positive attitude, optimism and being able to regulate your emotions— conveniently all things I'm going to talk about in this book, because these things are also related to boosting your self-esteem.

Here's the really good news: feeling great about yourself is a positive cycle. The better your self-esteem is, the better it continues to get—and the better everything else gets, too.

There's a bit of a stigma that loving yourself means you're conceited or 'up yourself', but I promise you that's just not true. Loving yourself is fantastic. It means you never let people treat you badly, it means you're confident, it means you enjoy your own company, and it's the only way to really maximise the potential to have a beautiful, fulfilling life. It's also the first step to truly loving other people, and cultivating strong, healthy relationships. And we all know we could all do with more of that in the world.

I'm sure you've heard the saying that to truly love someone else you have to love yourself first. We all say it, but how many of us *really* know what it means? How many of us put it into practice? Like anything, that saying's pretty open to interpretation, but when I compare relationships I've had in the past, when my self-esteem was low, to my relationship now, when my self-esteem is good, the difference is absolutely huge. When you have low self-esteem you can feel less deserving of happiness, and that can lead you to accept behaviour and treatment that is not OK in a relationship. In the past, when my self-esteem was low, I actually found myself *expecting* rejection (something I'm able to see now with the benefit of hindsight). I would overanalyse so many things and instantly put it down to the fact that my partner was rejecting me—'Oh, he's sick of me' or 'He's looking for someone better.' That simply meant that no amount of love from my partner was ever enough. I was trying to get love for myself from someone else, when it really needed to come from me. I just needed to love myself.

No matter how good our self-esteem is, we all need to practise a bit of self-love every now and then! It's just a really nice thing to do. Take a look at my self-love action plan over the page for some ideas you can start today.

TAKE CARE OF YOURSELF

At the same time as loving yourself, it's also important to take care of yourself—or, as people like to say these days, 'to practise self-care'. I'm sure you've heard a LOT of chat about self-care lately, as it's pretty trendy (which is fantastic, in my opinion). Basically, self-care is when you take action to preserve or improve your own health and well-being. Now, this doesn't just mean your physical health, but also your mental health, which is just as important.

Self-care is also about being gentle and kind to yourself. This means understanding from the outset that you're not perfect, and that's OK. (Perfection is not a thing, by the way. It simply doesn't exist.) It means

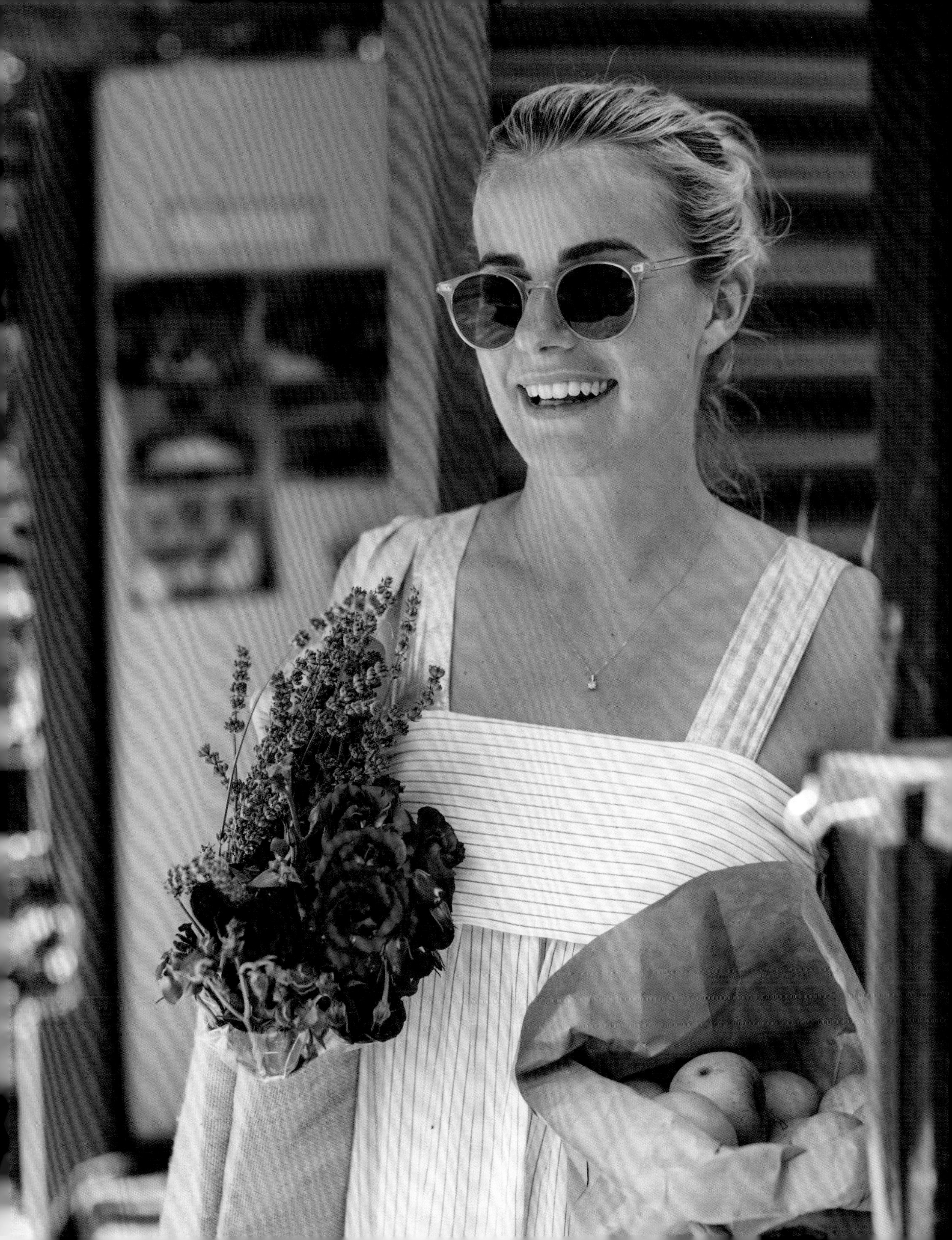

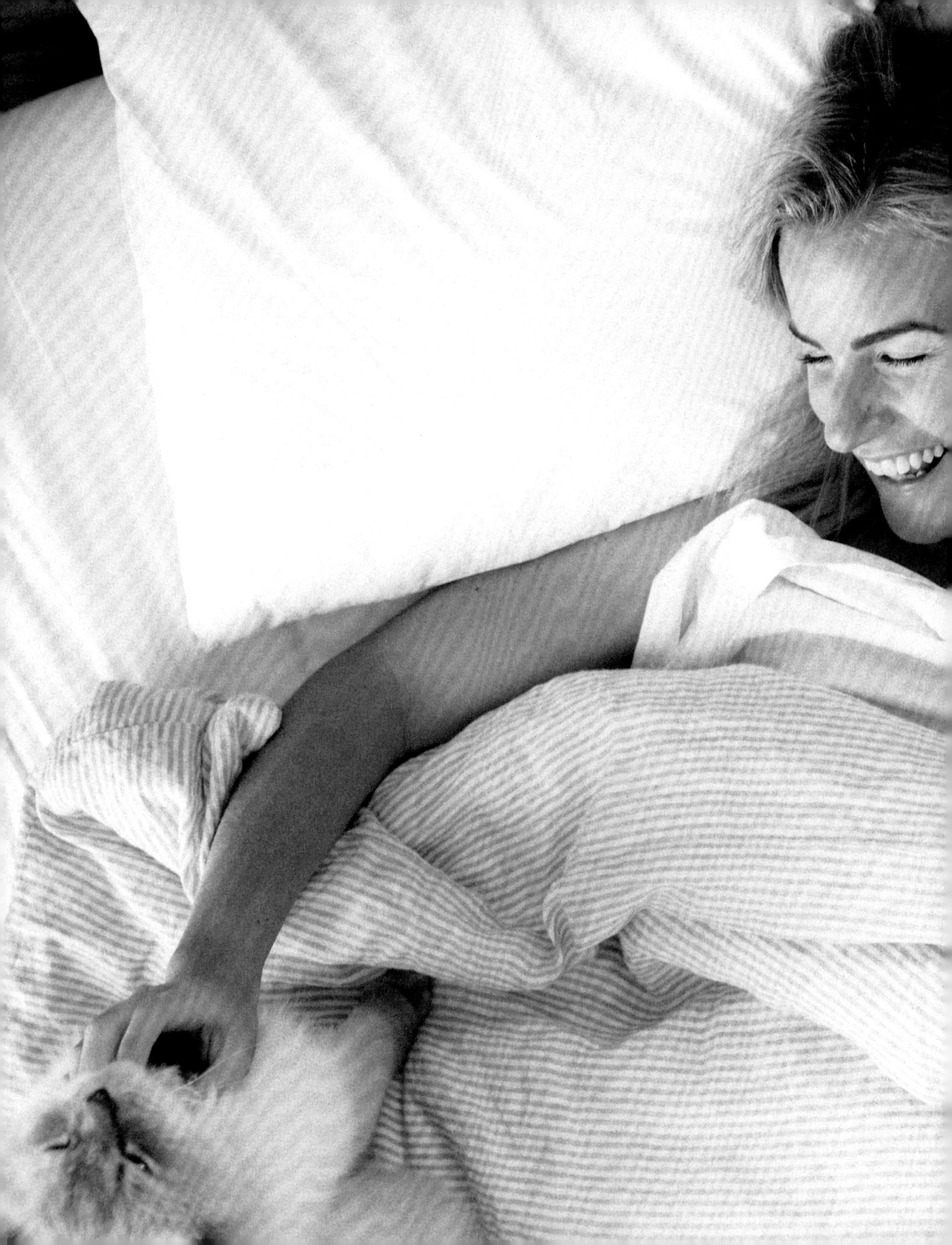

THE SELF-LOVE ACTION PLAN

* Remember that just because you think something about yourself, it doesn't mean it is true. Thinking and believing are two different things.

* Write down a compliment you receive. This may seem self-centred, but it's not. There's nothing wrong with remembering a compliment! We always seem to forget them so quickly, while insults stick in our minds like glue. It's important to try to change that.

* Check in with your own emotions. See how you're feeling each day, and don't judge yourself. Maybe you're feeling a little down, or you might be extraordinarily happy. Either way, just noting and acknowledging your emotions can be incredibly powerful. Sometimes, you might be grumpy for no reason. Learn to treat yourself with kindness. It's more than OK to feel that way.

* Learn to say no. I'm a recovering people-pleaser, so I struggle with this one. But it's really important to set your own boundaries and not take on too much at one time. You only have so much time and energy to give to others, and you need to remember to reserve some of that for yourself.

* Practise forgiveness. Holding on to grudges and resentment can be toxic for your well-being—emotionally and physically. Learn to forgive others, as well as yourself, and your soul will thank you for it. After all, you are only hurting yourself by holding on to it.

* Practise talking to yourself in the same way you would speak to a friend.

* Practise gratitude. (See Chapter Three on page 57.)

When you take care of yourself, it affirms your self-worth. By taking care of yourself and your needs, you're really telling yourself, 'I deserve this.' And it's true. You do.

acknowledging that you're trying to be a good person, even if you might not always get it a hundred per cent right. Try not to beat yourself up when you make mistakes or get things wrong. Instead, learn from those mistakes and use them to go forward as a bigger, braver, more open-minded person.

As I've already mentioned, looking after yourself goes hand in hand with your self-esteem. It's especially important to take care of yourself when things get tough, because strong self-esteem also makes *you* strong. It gives you resilience when life gets rocky. In July 2017, soon after developing Bell's palsy and having split from Brad Pitt, Angelina Jolie told *Vanity Fair*, 'Sometimes women in families put themselves last, until it manifests itself in their own health.' I love that quote. I also think the idea applies to everyone—if you don't take care of yourself, it's only a matter of time before that takes a toll on your body and your soul. You've probably heard the saying that you can't pour from an empty cup, and I couldn't agree with it more! The more you fill your own cup with self-love and self-care, the better placed you'll be to help fill the cups of others.

We live in such a fast-paced world that self-care is something we really have to choose, as it doesn't tend to be a part of our daily schedules unless we consciously make it so. We can easily get so caught up in our work, studies, families, social lives and everything else that we forget the importance of mental health. Self-care can be really beneficial when it comes to mental health, because it can have such a positive impact on your self-esteem. When you take care of yourself, it affirms your self-worth. By taking care of yourself and your needs, you're really telling yourself, 'I deserve this.' And it's true. You do.

However, there is sometimes a bit of a misconception out there that self-care is 'elitist' because it costs a lot of money and is only for people who have a heap of free time. True self-care doesn't have to cost a cent! And it doesn't have to mean going to a spa for hours, either. It can be as simple as putting on your favourite song and having a five-minute dance party all by yourself.

Do you know what else? When you take care of yourself, it encourages your friends and family to look after themselves too. If that's not a good thing, I don't know what is. We are all constantly learning from each other, after all.

If you pay attention, you'll notice your body tells you when it's time for a little bit of self-care. The message can manifest in many ways. I first learnt what self-care was a couple of years back, when I was experiencing this intense brain fog from floating around with no purpose. I had just started a business that I didn't really believe in simply to have an excuse to leave my old job, but I just ended up feeling lost and aimless. I realised the mental fog I was battling was a result of the fact that I had no idea what I was doing with my life! I decided I needed to take better care of myself—not just in the sense of exercise and nutrition (although that was part of it), but also in my head, so to speak.

For others, the message might be delivered by your body getting sick or feeling exhausted. You might feel like you've got no time for yourself. You might even just plain feel like shit. I hear you. There's often a good reason for these sorts of feelings. Lots of us don't realise, until we really take a step back to assess things, just how much we're trying to do and how many things we're trying to be for others. We're trying to spin so many other people's plates for them that we forget about our own. Well, maybe you just need to let those other people take care of their own plates for a bit, while you make sure yours don't break.

When I first started out on my own self-care journey, I didn't really have any idea what to do. I just knew I needed to do something. So, I decided to give the whole self-care thing a go and just see what happened. And you know what? It was so good that I still practise self-care today. Plus, the benefit of me learning about self-care is that I've got a bunch of tips to share. That means you don't need to start from scratch. Who doesn't love a shortcut?

I hope that, after reading this chapter, you have more of an understanding about what self-love and self-care really are, and why they're such important building blocks for good self-esteem. The tips in the action plans are simple, you can do them every day and they don't have to cost money. The main takeaway here is to start prioritising yourself every once in a while.

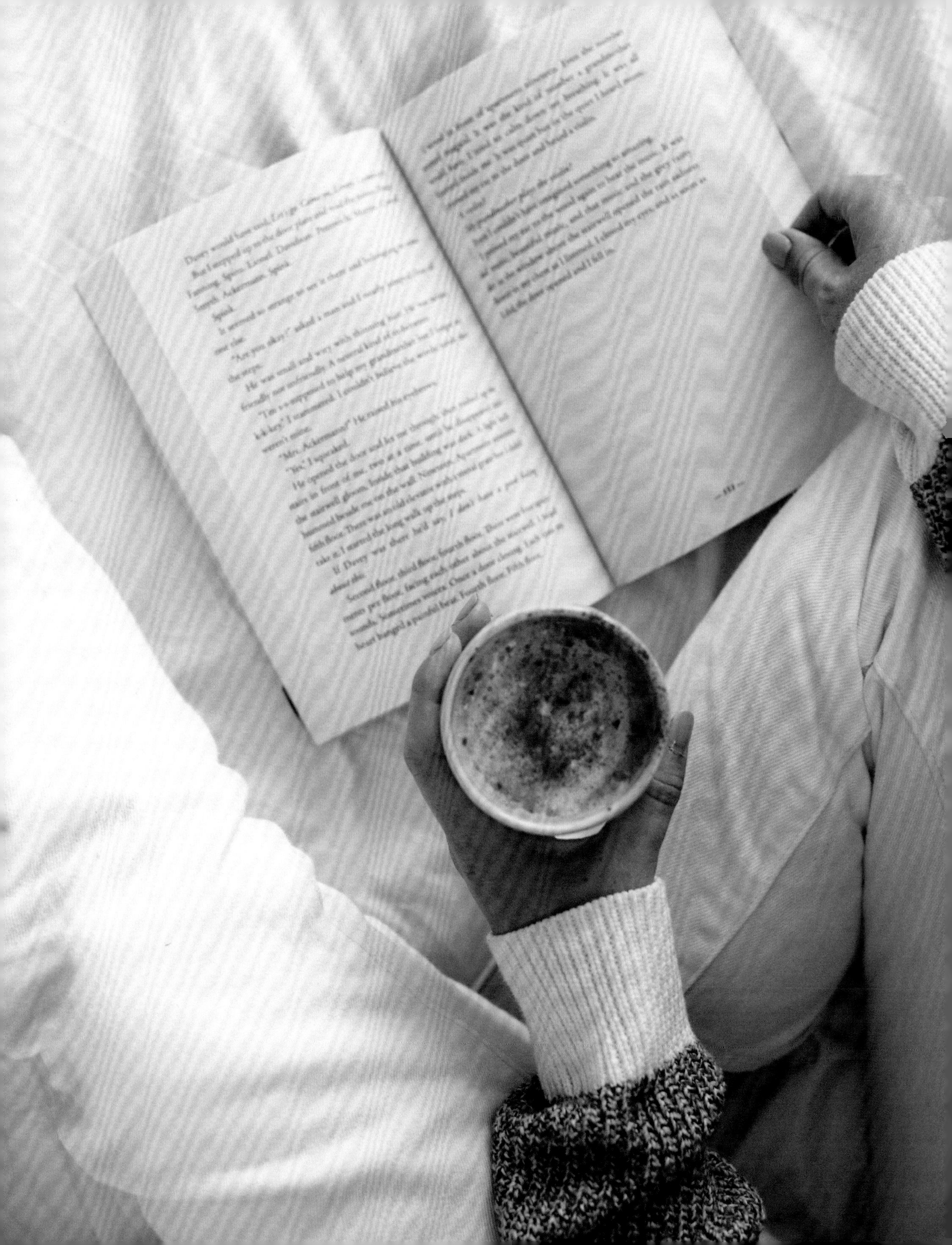

THE SELF-CARE ACTION PLAN

* Get away from screens for an hour a day. Screens will suck out our souls if we let them! They can stifle creativity and are huge time-wasters if we don't set boundaries. Just taking an hour to get away from them and do something else, like go out for a coffee or a walk, can do wonders for the soul.

* If you have a pet, spend a bit of time every day just hanging out with them. It can be easy to overlook your furry friends, but they bring so much joy! I'm sure they love it when they feel appreciated too. Also, you are basically your pet's whole world. They are your biggest fan, which can give you a little boost after a tough day. (Unless you have cats, like I do. Sometimes I'm not sure if my cats even know who I am, but I like to think they love me as much as I love them . . .)

* Be a bit selfish. Even if it's just for ten minutes. Do something for you. Run a bath instead of having a quick shower, watch your favourite show even if everyone else hates it, paint your nails, make yourself your favourite treat . . . You get the picture. It's important to take the time to treat yourself—and just yourself.

* Spend time outside. I know when I'm a little stressed or out of sorts, I become somewhat of a hermit! I don't do a lot of exercise and just stay inside my little stress cave thinking about how stressed I am. But, as soon as I get outside for a walk or a jog or even just to sit on my back deck for 20 minutes or so, I instantly feel better. Nature has an incredible effect on the soul.

* Hydrate yoself! Drink lots more water. Your skin, energy levels and digestive system will thank you for it.

> >

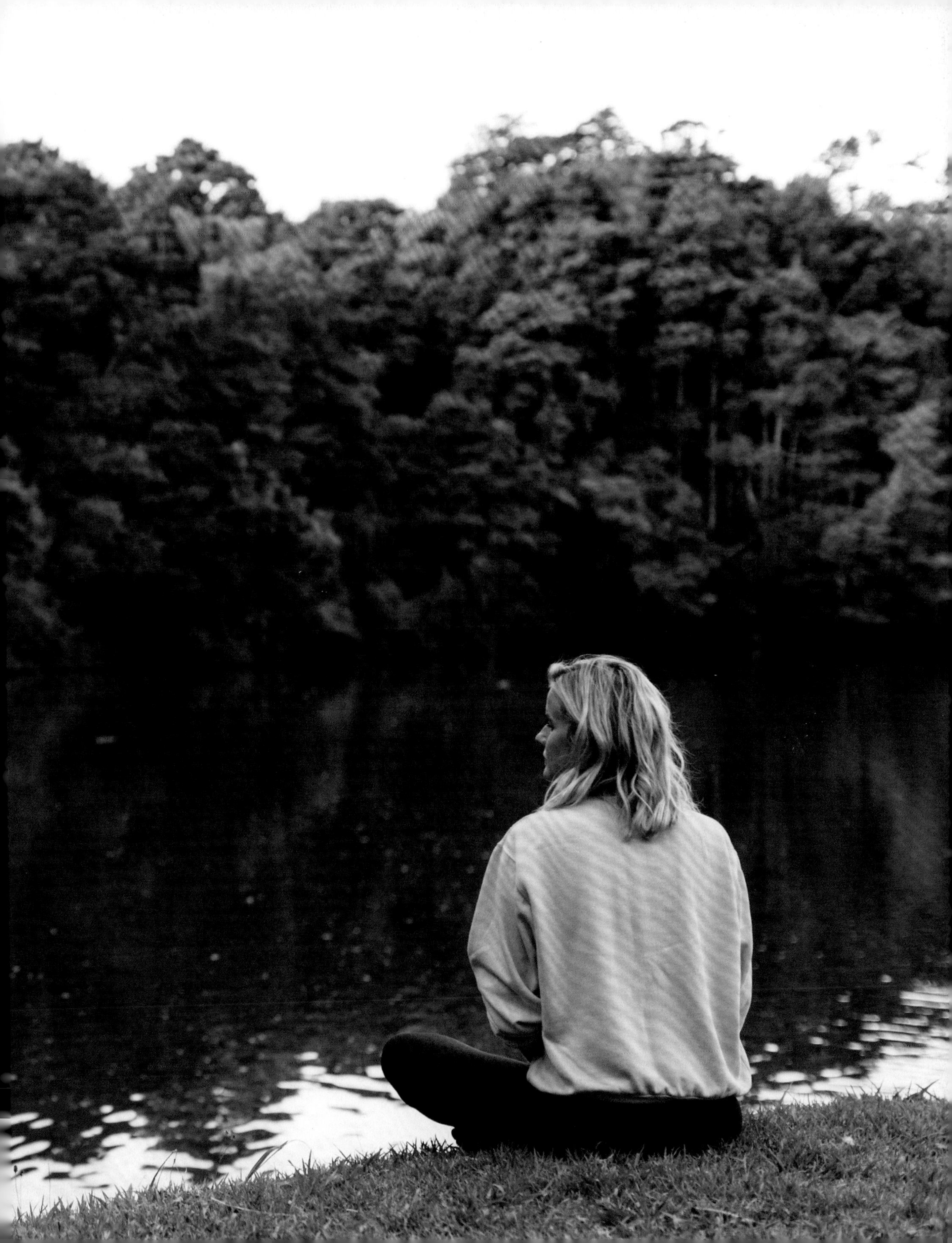

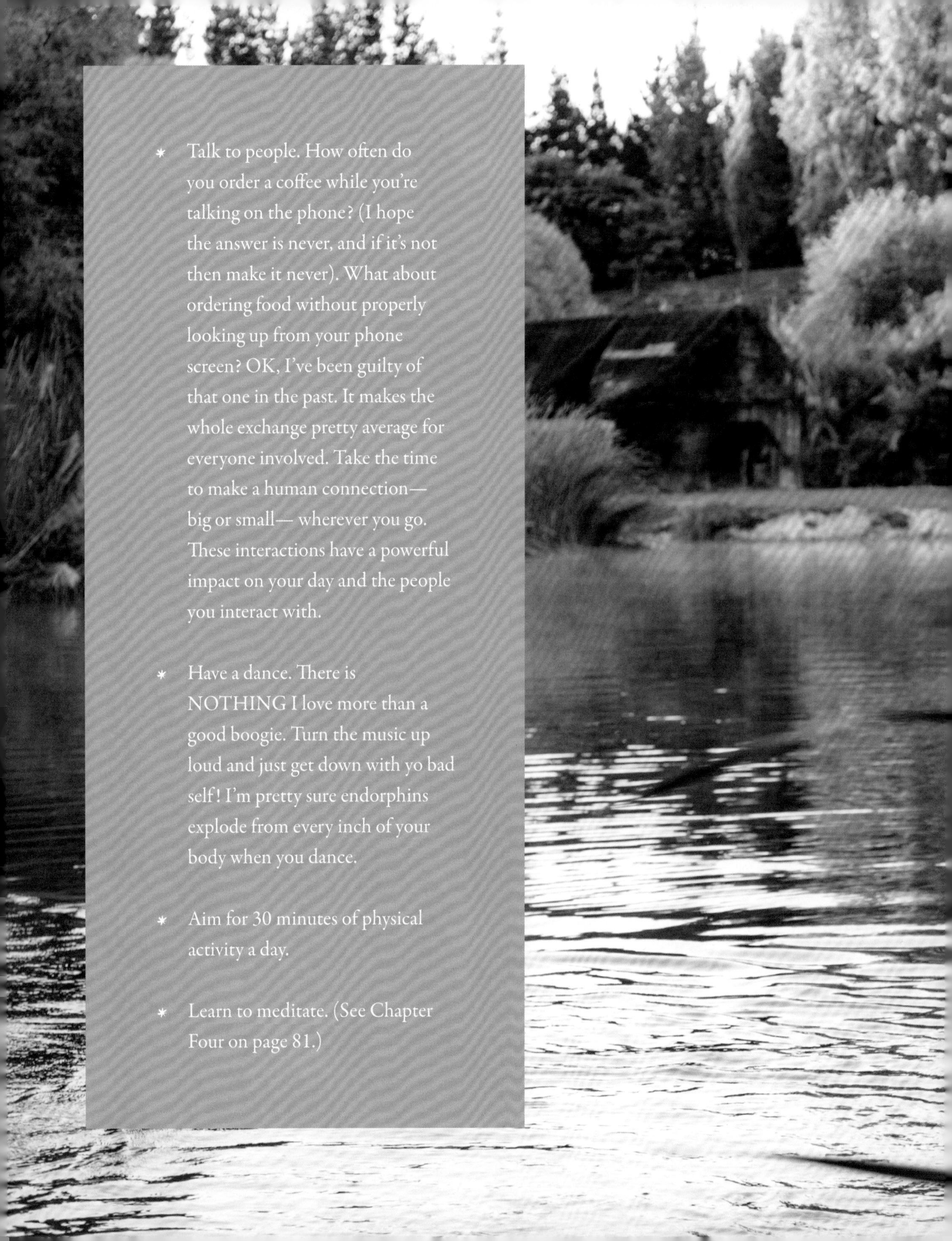

* Talk to people. How often do you order a coffee while you're talking on the phone? (I hope the answer is never, and if it's not then make it never). What about ordering food without properly looking up from your phone screen? OK, I've been guilty of that one in the past. It makes the whole exchange pretty average for everyone involved. Take the time to make a human connection— big or small— wherever you go. These interactions have a powerful impact on your day and the people you interact with.

* Have a dance. There is NOTHING I love more than a good boogie. Turn the music up loud and just get down with yo bad self! I'm pretty sure endorphins explode from every inch of your body when you dance.

* Aim for 30 minutes of physical activity a day.

* Learn to meditate. (See Chapter Four on page 81.)

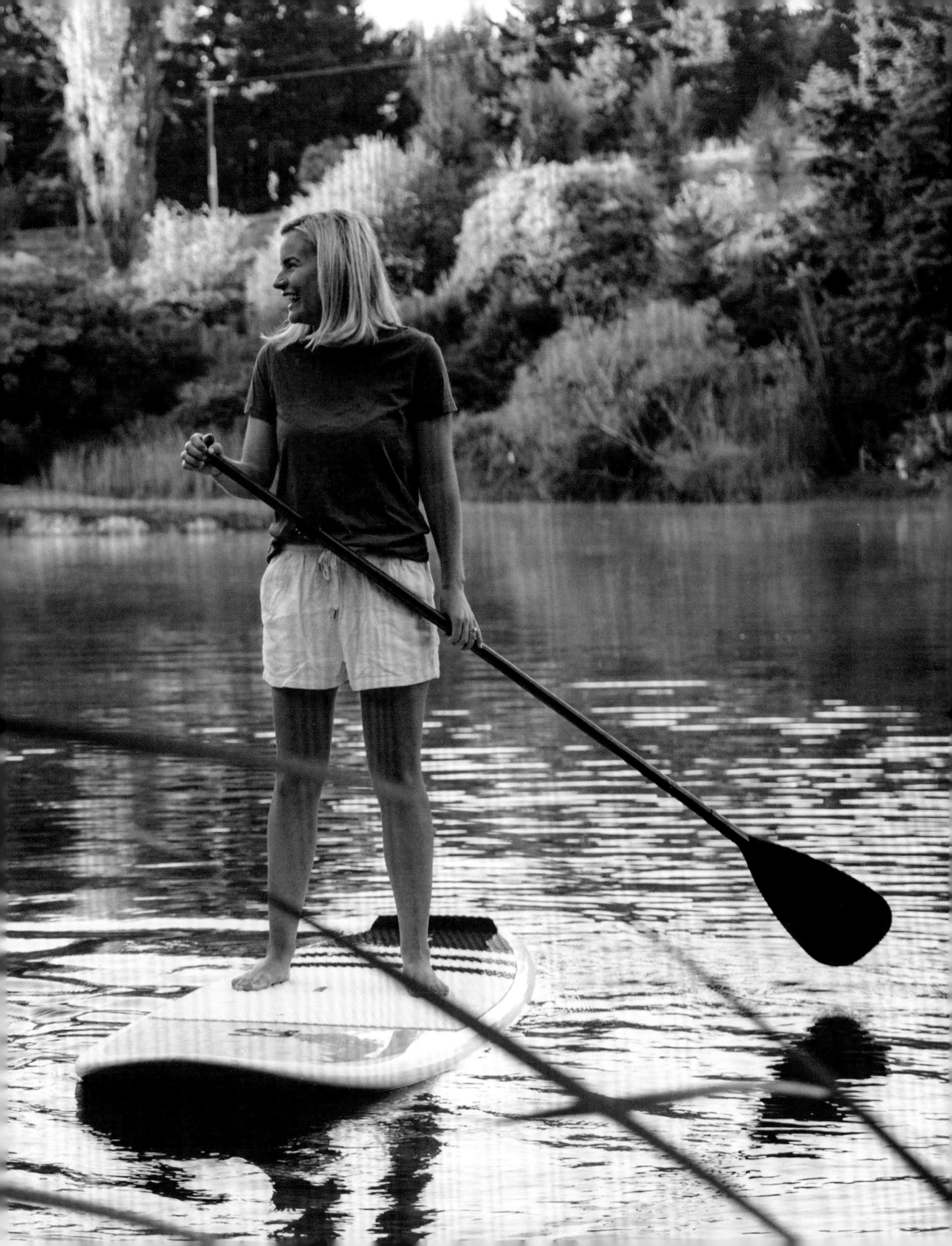

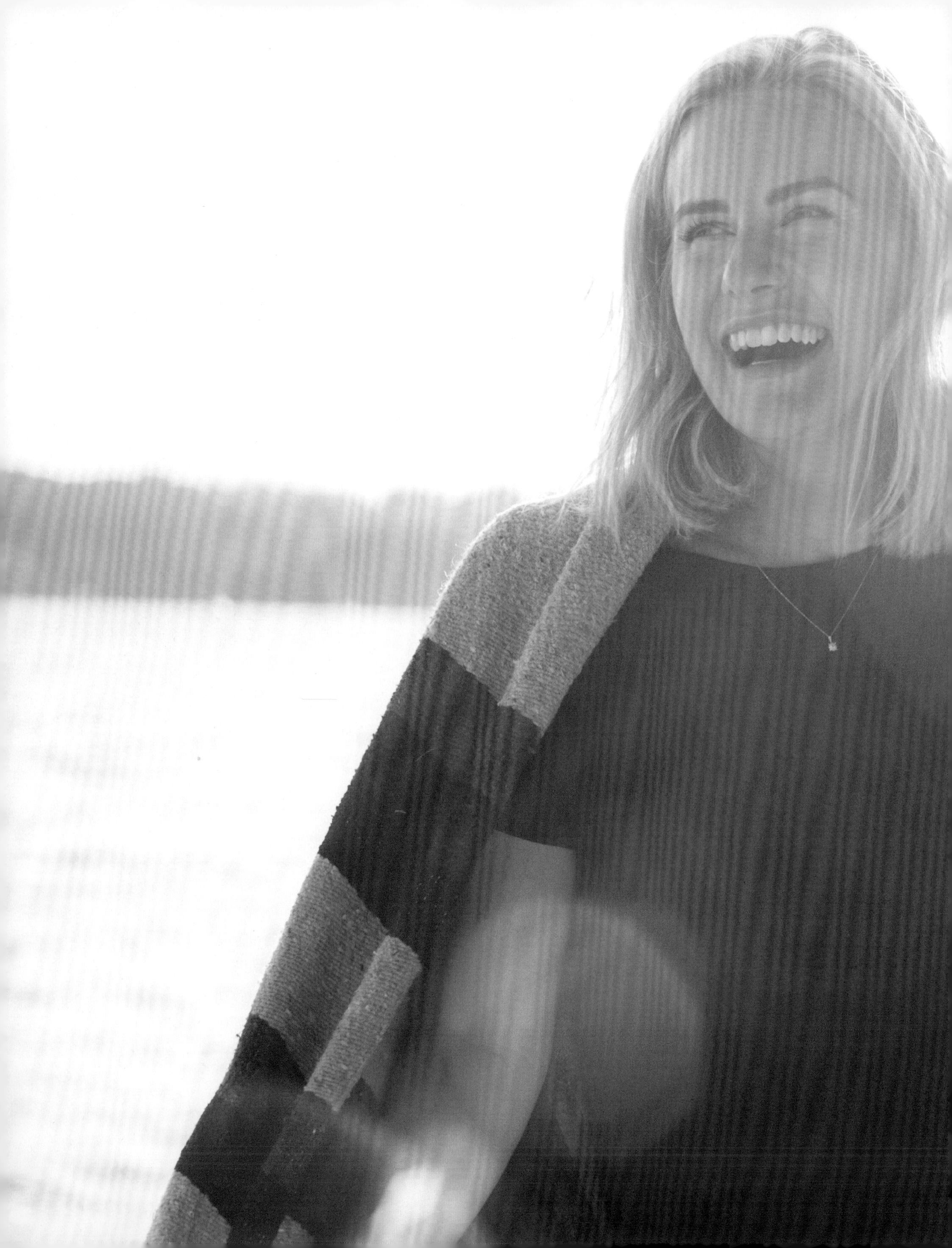

Chapter Three

GRATITUDE

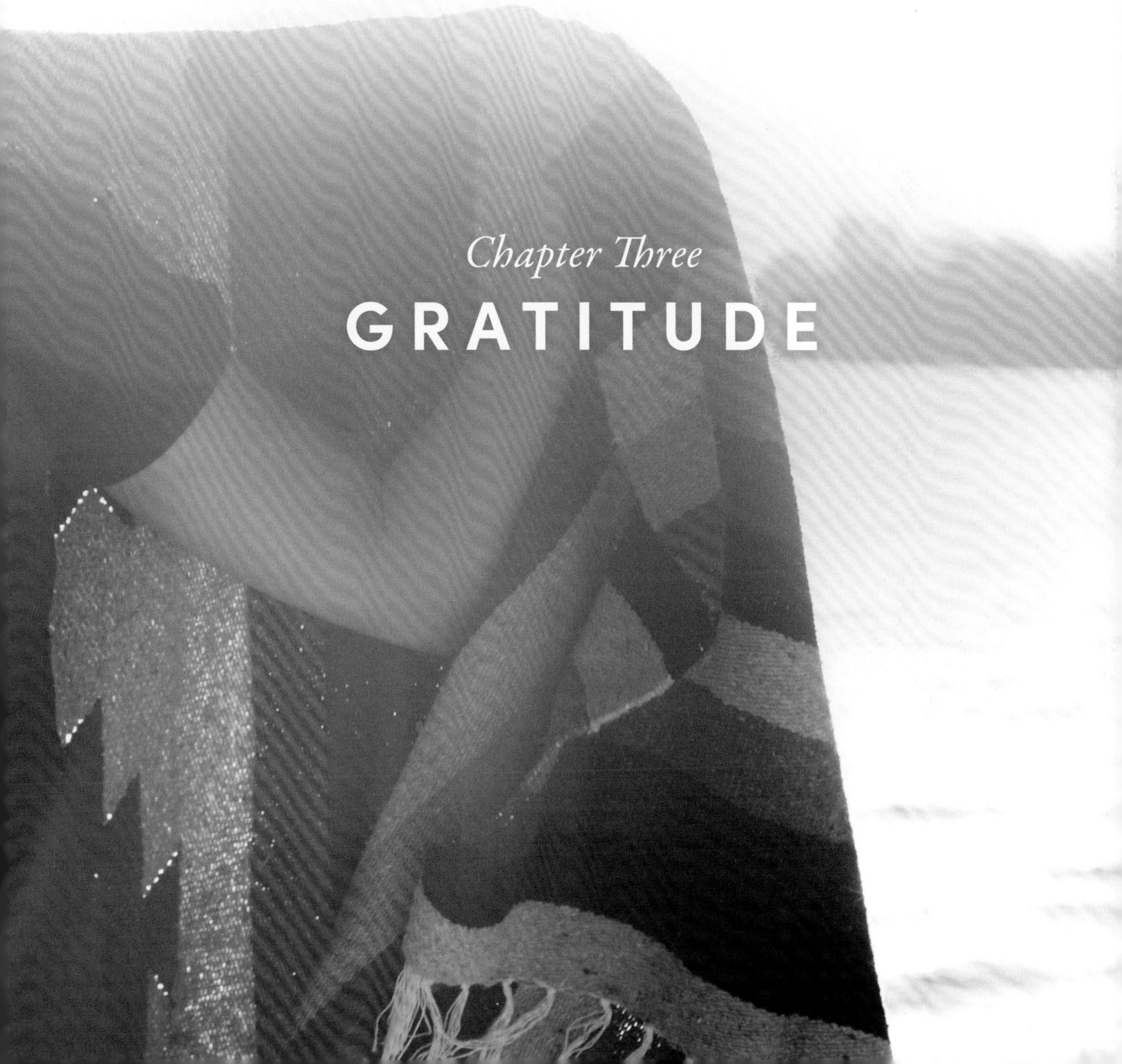

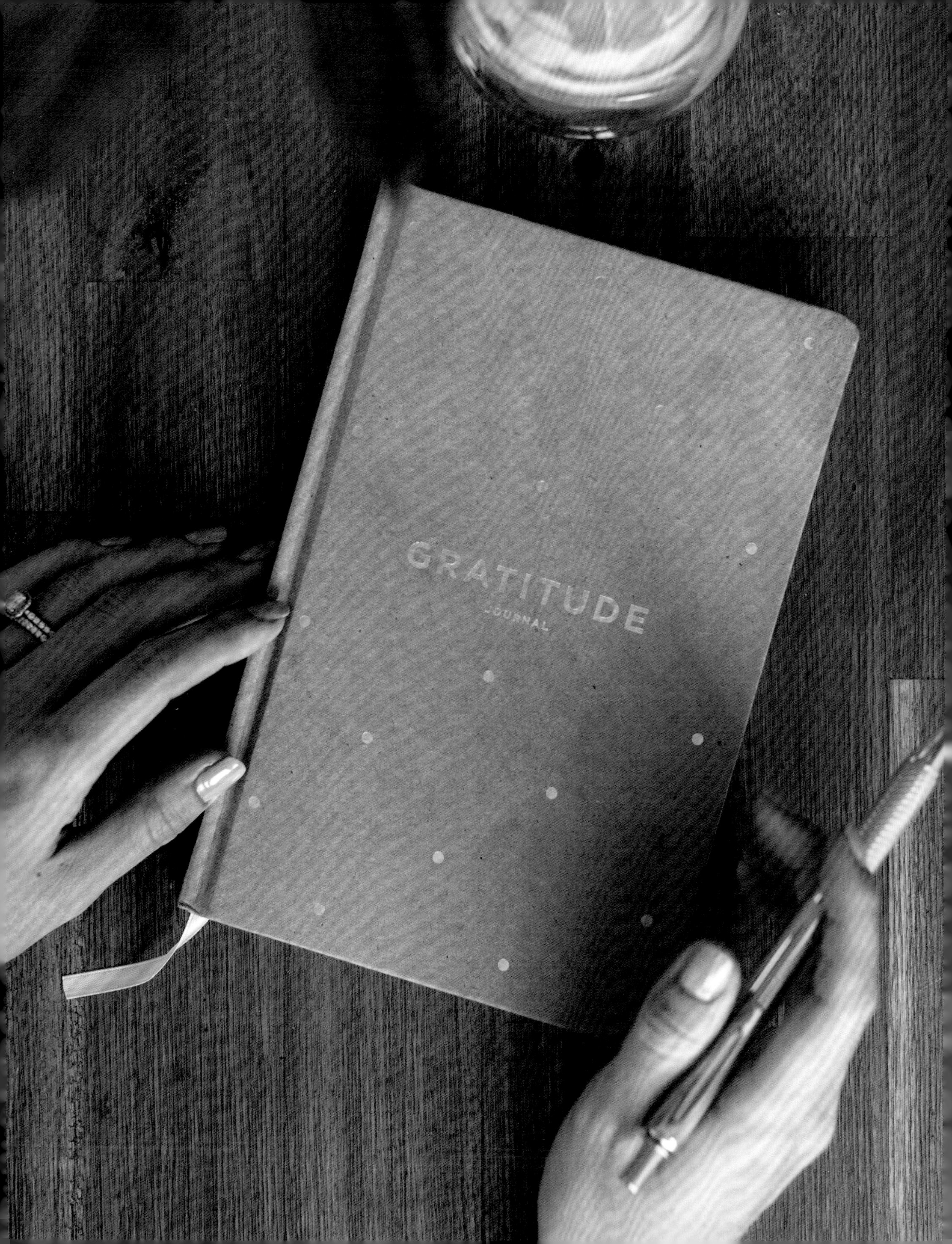
GRATITUDE
JOURNAL

So, we've covered the basics of self-esteem, and some of the things (good and bad) that affect it? Tick. And we've talked about why it's important to start from a solid foundation of self-love and self-care? Tick. Cool! In that case, I reckon we can get started on the really good stuff—all the tips and tricks I know to take your self-esteem to the next level. As I've said, these are just some suggestions based on personal experience. I'm hoping all the things I've learnt over the last couple of years will help you too.

The first concept I'm going to talk about is one you've probably already heard of: gratitude. Chances are, you've seen #gratitude popping up all over your Instagram feed, or you've heard people chatting about it here and there. You might already know all about it (in which case, this chapter's just going to be covering old territory for you, isn't it, smarty pants?). If you're one of the uninitiated, you a) might not care what gratitude is or b) may have caught yourself wondering more than once what it really means. Is it just feeling grateful for things? Is it about getting more things in your life to feel grateful for? What things are we even talking about? Why does it even matter, this feeling grateful business? It sounds a bit wishy-washy, to be honest . . .

If this is you, I'm just going to stop you right there for a gosh darn second. We're going to take it right back to square one.

WHAT EVEN IS GRATITUDE?

So, let's begin with that idea of 'more', because it's actually pretty relevant here. In today's world, it can often seem like everything is all about getting 'more'. We want 'more money', 'more clothes', 'more friends', 'more followers'—you name it, someone wants more of it. No matter what we have, it never seems to ever be enough.

'But what does gratitude have to do with any of that?' I hear you ask. Good question! And one that conveniently brings us to our next point of discussion: what gratitude is. In really super-duper basic terms, gratitude is the practice of feeling grateful for aspects of your current life. The word 'practice' is a pretty key one there, because gratitude is exactly that. A practice. It's something you have to make an effort to do, day after day after day.

I'm going to hand over to an expert here for a moment, so we can really zero in on what gratitude is and make sure it's crystal clear. Dr Robert A. Emmons is a leading researcher in gratitude at the University of California, Davis, and he has a two-pronged definition of gratitude that does a very good job of defining it. (I believe that's why he's an expert.)

* First, he calls gratitude 'an affirmation of goodness'—which is to say, it's an acknowledgement that the world and our lives do contain good things. He's careful to point out that this doesn't mean that life is perfect, or doesn't also contain bad bits. Gratitude, he says, simply 'encourages us to identify some amount of goodness in our life'.

* Second, he says practising gratitude involves working out where the good stuff comes from. Importantly, he points out that we should recognise the good stuff that comes from outside of our selves.

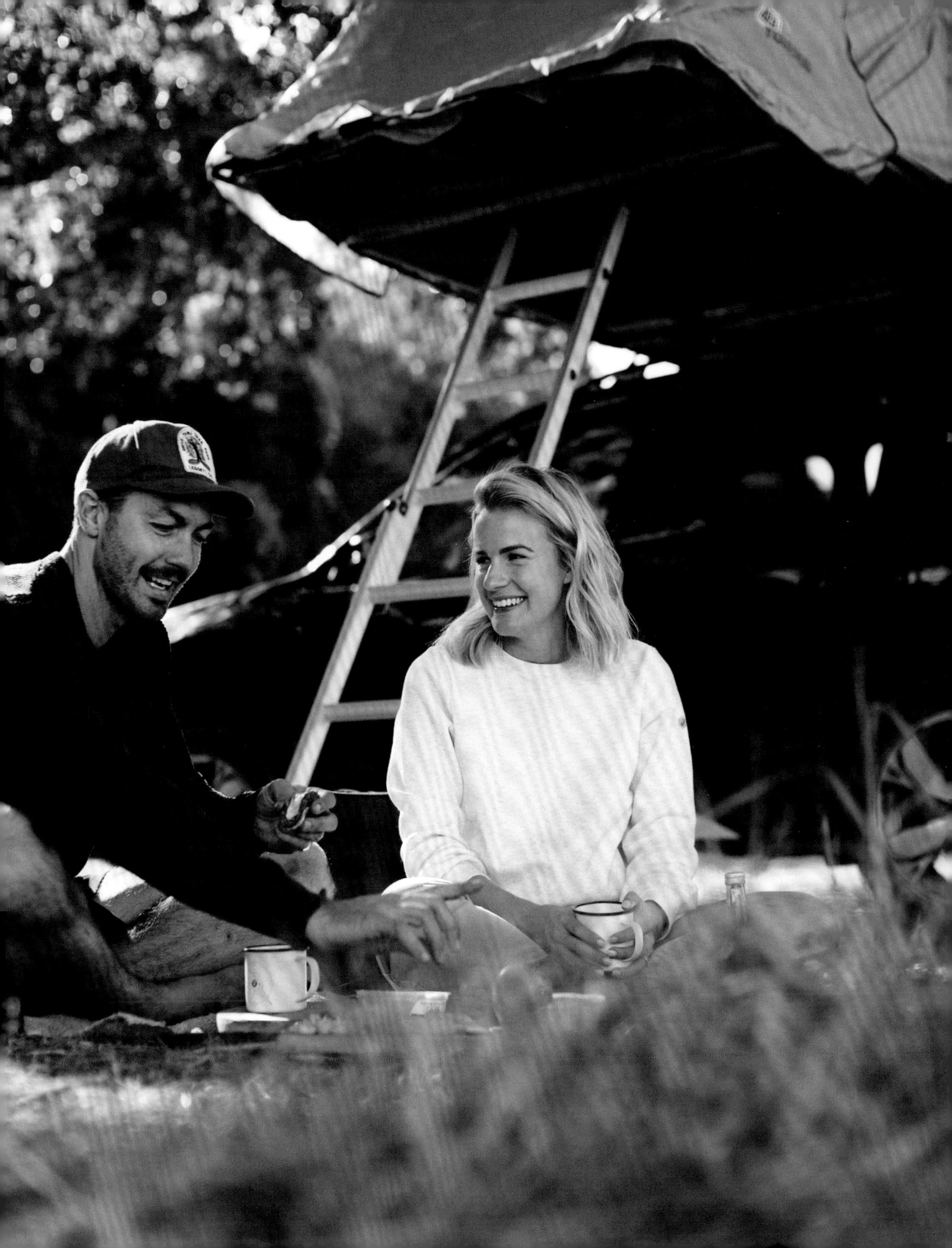

More positive emotions?
Fewer negative ones? Makes
you tougher, and also helps
you feel pretty good about
yourself? Who *wouldn't* want
more of that in their lives?

'Well, that's all lovely and stuff,' you might now be saying, 'but why bother? What's the point?'

Our very smart pal Rob has already beaten you to that one. In a 2010 article he wrote for University of California, Berkeley's *Greater Good Magazine* called 'Why Gratitude Is Good', he explained that gratitude does four important things: it magnifies positive emotions, it blocks negative ones (like envy, resentment and regret), it makes us more resilient and stress-resistant, and it improves our self-esteem.

More positive emotions? Fewer negative ones? Makes you tougher, and also helps you feel pretty good about yourself? Who *wouldn't* want more of that in their lives? Sign me up!

GRATITUDE AND ME

I first heard about gratitude a few years ago when Instagram was becoming a thing. It was mainly the spiritual yogis I followed who were talking about it so, to be honest, I kind of just wrote it off as a spiritual yogi thing . . . I believed I was much further away from that sort of mindset than I actually was. I'll be the first to put my hand up and say I only got into practising gratitude when it became more mainstream. Yes, I'm one of those ones. But, as soon as I started, I was well and truly sold.

At the time I started practising gratitude, I remember feeling a little all over the place and highly strung, as if my brain was a bit scrambled. I was also craving some form of creativity, although I didn't realise it then. So, how do I feel now, after practising it for a while? Well, I've actually noticed quite a few positive changes. I can handle stress far better, I no longer go through life taking everything for granted, I'm far more self-assured and secure in who I am, and I even feel like I'm much more creative.

It really has had such a profound effect on me personally. When I first started, I had to sit up and think, *Well, OK . . . There has to be something in this right?* Now, I try to practise some form of gratitude every day—but I'm only human, so I do come and go with it a bit. Sometimes I'll have stages where I practise it lots, and other times, when 'life gets in the way', I don't do it as much. The key, as with everything, is to just do what works for you. I try not to be too hard on myself, and just fit it in when I'm able to.

THE GLASS IS HALF FULL

OK, so hopefully you're now starting to get a clearer picture of how gratitude can be a bloody useful tool to building good self-esteem and a more fulfilled life. It sounds airy-fairy, but until you actively practise it on a regular basis it's hard to understand what kind of effect it can have. As I've mentioned, I've enjoyed so many benefits from practising gratitude. I hope you'll consider giving it a go, too.

Just in case you're still not totally sold on the idea, let's take a closer look at some of the main benefits and how they can actually manifest when you make gratitude a habit. First up, optimism and positive emotions! Regularly practising gratitude can help to make you more optimistic than pessimistic. I believe that people naturally lean more towards either positivity or negativity, but I also believe that's something that can be changed with some self-awareness and effort thrown in.

Personally, I'm more drawn to the positive, but that doesn't mean I'm positive about everything. I have my days when everything seems to be going wrong and I feel like the world is against me. Those are the days when practising gratitude really comes in handy. Gratitude focuses on the good in life, and if we perceive our current life to have more good, we will also perceive our future life to have more good. (I'm not sure if that makes grammatical sense, but let's go with it.) I guess, in a way, that's what hope is.

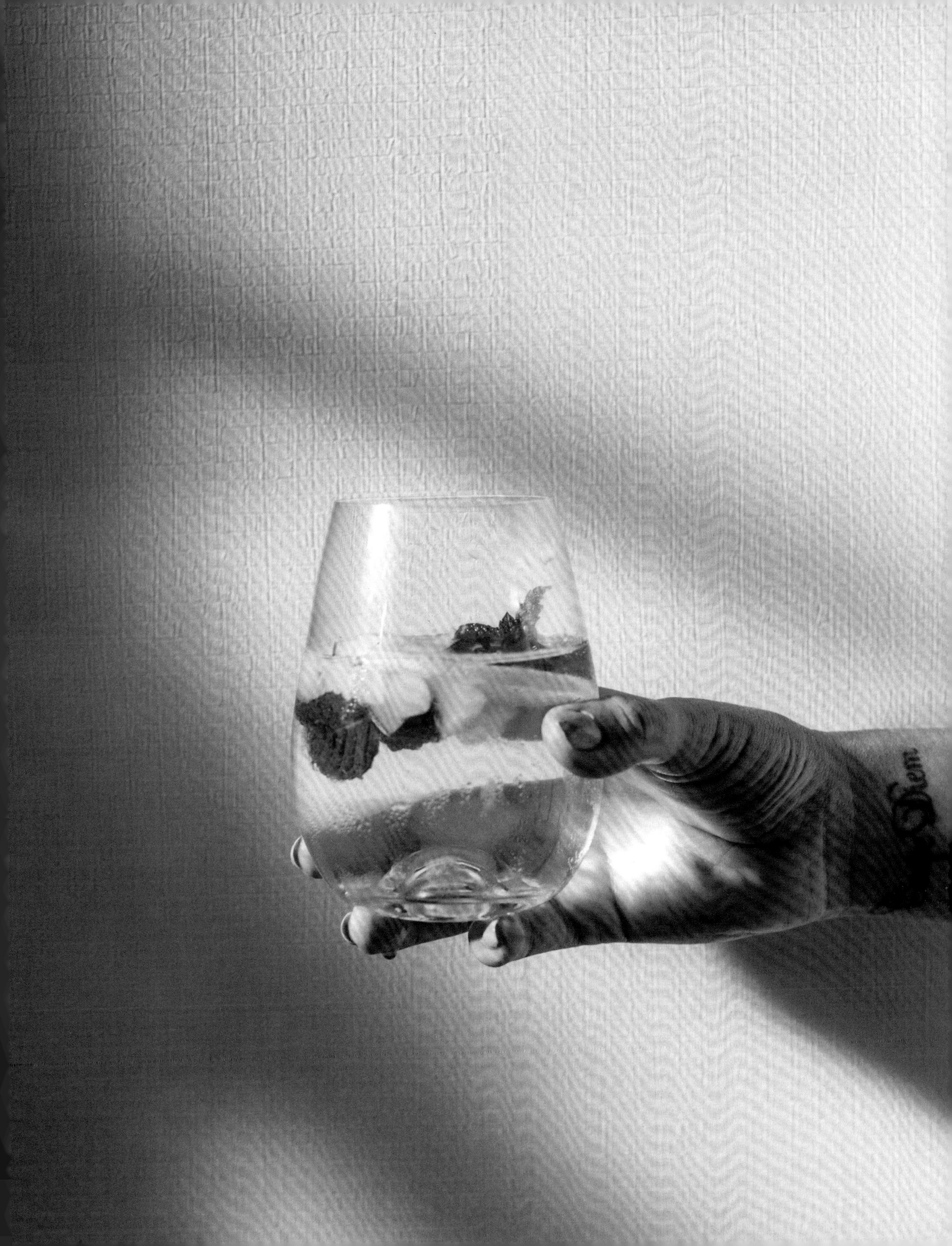

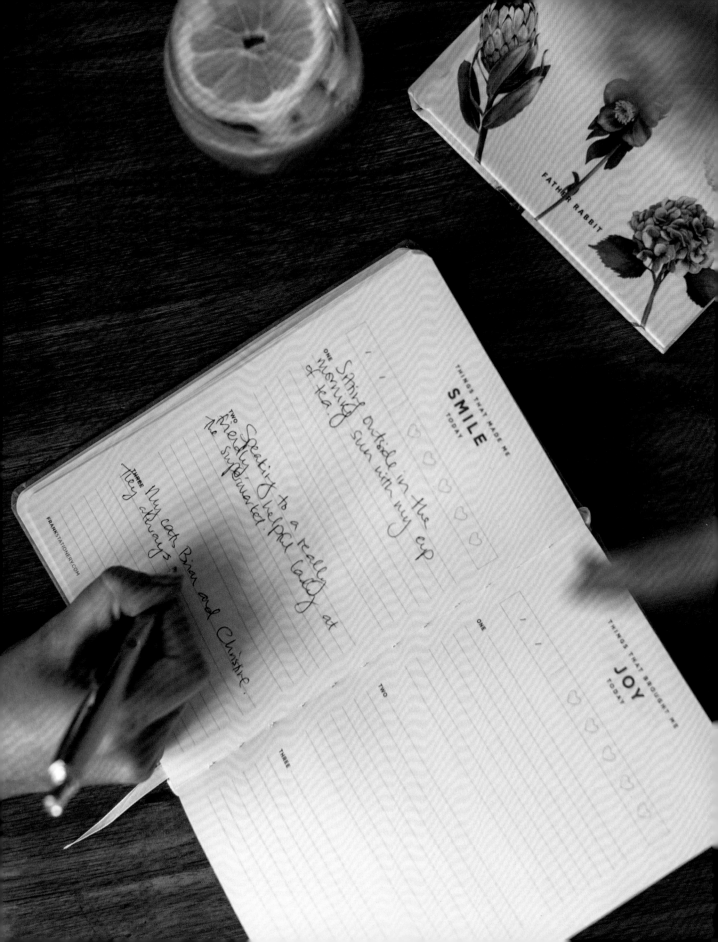

THINGS THAT MADE ME
SMILE
TODAY

ONE Sitting outside in the morning sun with my cup of tea.

TWO Speaking to a really friendly & helpful lady at the supermarket.

THREE My cats Brian and Christine. They always

THINGS THAT BROUGHT ME
JOY
TODAY

ONE

TWO

THREE

FRANKSTATIONERY.COM

FATHER RABBIT

And hope is the perfect thing to cling to when the world feels big and scary.

I know lots of people think hope is a bit of a pushover emotion—sort of like gratitude, come to think of it—but you know what? I think hope can be pretty profound (and so do lots of other people). It's a brave thing to hope for better in the world, even if the world doesn't seem to be giving you many examples of good things. And, let me ask you this: if we aren't hoping for better—and, as a result, also trying to make our own little worlds better by being better ourselves—then what hope is there? Some people like to poo-poo positivity and hope because they think that hopeful and positive people are naive, but I don't believe that's true. I think the world needs more hopeful, positive people, so why not be one of them yourself?

BYE-BYE, BAD FEELINGS

Many of us are already all too aware, from personal experience, of how negative thoughts and toxic mind-chatter can hurt us. You know the toxic mind-chatter I'm talking about, don't you? Doubting yourself, feeling insecure about certain things, feeling guilty, feeling afraid and so on. Thoughts that sound like *I'm never going to be good at this so I'm going to give up now* or *I'll probably fail this class as I'm not smart enough* or *I don't want to exercise because I'm embarrassed and people will stare at me.*

When left unchecked and unaddressed, these sorts of thoughts can wreak havoc on our inner selves. We don't tend to realise it, but our world can start to revolve around this sort of toxic mind-chatter and any related negative feelings. Things can easily spiral out of control, resulting in anything from missed opportunities we were too scared to grasp to staying in unhealthy relationships because we think it's all we deserve.

Gratitude can start to turn these negative feelings around, as it's impossible to be thinking negative thoughts while practising gratitude. The whole point is to start to appreciate the people and the world around you, connect on a deeper level with yourself, and in turn gain a whole new level of acceptance towards yourself. Gratitude also helps you notice the good that is all around you, so that's what you start to focus on instead of the bad. When these positive feelings and thoughts get bigger and more common, there's simply less room for the negative.

I find that gratitude helps me to focus on the present moment, instead of stressing about the past or the future. It helps me to appreciate where I'm at in life. This is important because, sometimes, we can get so caught up in our goals and working towards them that we forget to stop, take a breath, turn around and admire the view.

GET GRATITUDE TOUGH

Life is not always plain sailing. There are highs, there are lows, happy days and sad days. Before I found the power of gratitude, I would just take these as they came, letting the emotion of everything completely consume me. I didn't feel as though I had any control over anything. If I was going through a tough time, I felt like it was happening 'to me'.

Gratitude has helped me to build my own resilience, and I now know how powerful that can really be. How does gratitude make you more resilient? Well, I've already mentioned how gratitude helps to keep you grounded and in the moment, but also starts to make you more hopeful and optimistic, right? Well, I think that's what does it.

If you practise gratitude when times are good, you are much more prepared for the times when things aren't so great. I don't feel like a victim of circumstance when times are tough any more. Now, I feel like I can face challenges head on and also appreciate how they will make me a better person in the long run.

We can get so caught up
in our goals and working
towards them that we forget
to stop, take a breath, turn
around and admire the view.

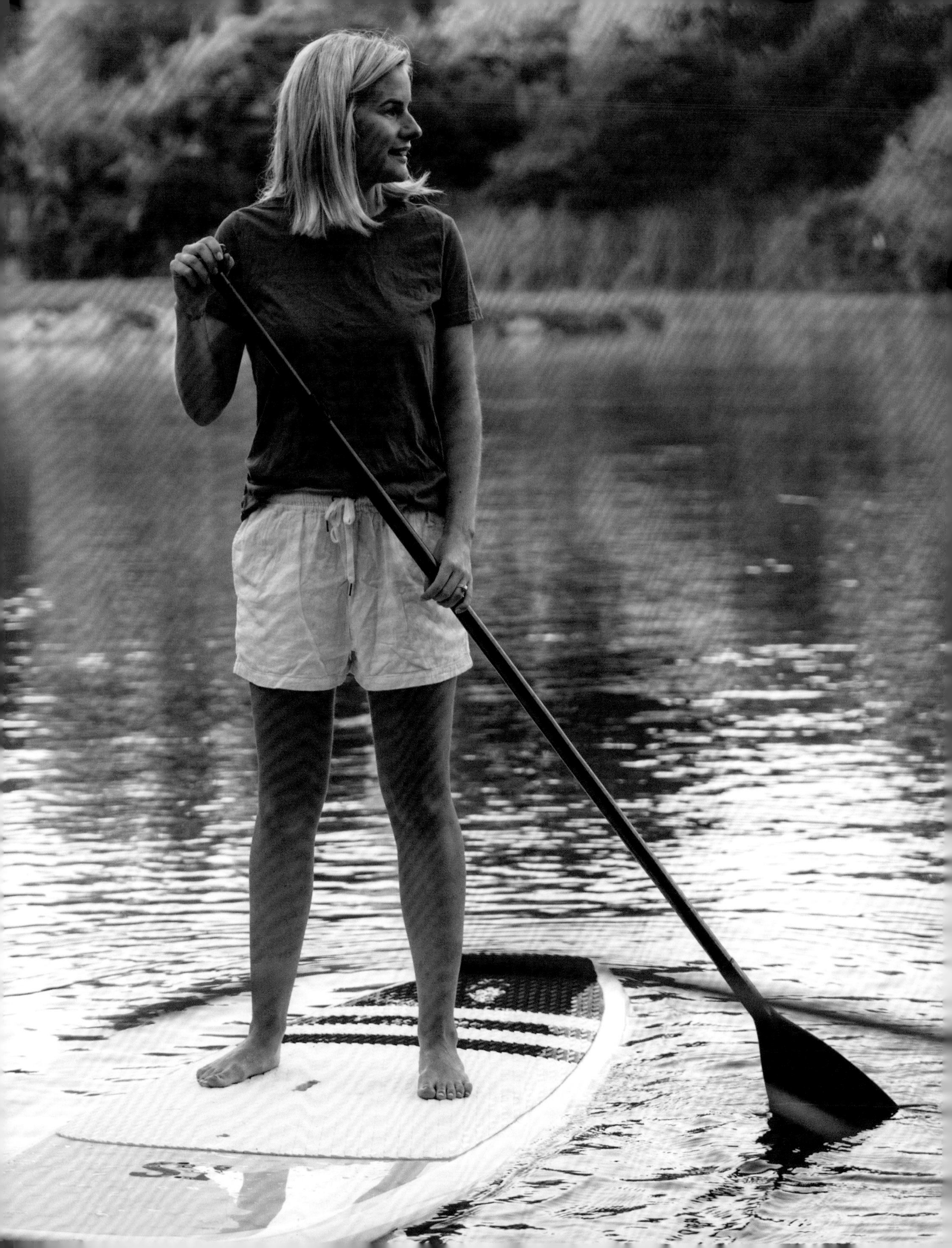

TAKE A LOOK AROUND YOU

Another happy side effect of gratitude is that it encourages us to think of others.

I can't tell you the number of times I've heard the phrase 'me me me' thrown around in the same sentence as 'social media' (mainly from the baby boomer generation, to be honest), and I have to agree that social media can have the potential to make us a little self-obsessed. Social media, by its very nature, is the act of sharing your life with others, so there's a lot of talking about yourself. There's not necessarily anything wrong with that (actually, I think we could all do with singing our own praises a bit more!), but I do think it's important to be aware of it, and keep a balance. The more you practise gratitude and start to appreciate others and the world around you a little more, the easier maintaining that balance will become.

Improving your self-esteem is a journey inward, but practising gratitude can help balance that by focusing your attention outward. And, in the process of focusing on yourself less, you can actually better your self-esteem! Lots of people have bad self-esteem because, paradoxically, they're concentrating way too hard on themselves. They're scrutinising every little thing about their bodies, lives, friends, social media feeds . . . and in the process forgetting to look up and around them and pay a bit more attention to others. Part of feeling good about yourself is actually not looking too hard at yourself—it's just accepting all the wonderful things you have to offer, and leaving it at that.

Also, when you take the time to appreciate others, you can start to see the things in yourself that other people appreciate about YOU. It's all about getting a bit of perspective and being grateful for other people in your life— their smiles, their support, their humour, their generosity. All of these things help make us more empathetic, more understanding of others, and this in turn humbles us.

How does 'being humble' tie in to self-esteem, you ask? Well, I think the people with the strongest sense of self-esteem are so happy within themselves

When you are humble, you stop trying to always beat everyone. Instead, you let other people be themselves—at the same time as letting you be yourself.

that they don't feel like they have anything to prove. People with good self-esteem recognise their strengths, but also recognise that they have weaknesses and that's totally OK. When you are humble, you stop trying to always beat everyone. Instead, you let other people be themselves—at the same time as letting you be yourself.

GET ON THE GRATITUDE TRAIN

I think I've shown you by now just how good gratitude is for us, but if that's not enough let's bring some science into the mix. Study after study has shown the various and wide-ranging benefits a gratitude practice can bring to our lives.

As an article published in 2018 in *Greater Good Magazine* noted, 'the evidence is mounting that gratitude may well be one of the fundamental pillars of a healthy lifestyle'. In 2015, *Psychology Today* published '7 Scientifically Proven Benefits of Gratitude', and listed research that has shown just some of the ways gratitude is good for us—namely, it opens the door to more relationships, improves our physical and psychological health, enhances our empathy and reduces aggression, makes us sleep better, boosts our self-esteem and even increases our mental strength. That's a bunch of good stuff right there, that is.

Right now, there's this amazing movement that has 'positive psychology' at its heart, and gratitude fits right in. In a 2003 paper called 'Counting blessings versus burdens', psychology researchers from University of California, Davis, documented a study in which a group of subjects kept a personal journal for ten weeks. In the journal, they rated their mood, physical health and other factors that contribute to being happy. They were told to either describe five things they were grateful for that had occurred in the past week (the gratitude condition), or they did the opposite and described five daily hassles that they were displeased about (the hassles condition). Researchers found that those in the gratitude group reported fewer health complaints and even spent more time exercising than the control participants did. Pretty cool, right? I really love that people who are far more academic than I am are taking the time to research things that have previously been written off as 'hippy stuff'.

So, there you have it. Gratitude is not just some wishy-washy spiritual-yogi thing. It's simply something that can be really good for your lifestyle and your mind.

One last thing: gratitude is a gradual process. Think of it as like going to the gym for your brain. Over time, you will train your brain so it starts to use its positive neural pathways by default more often. Basically, you'll naturally be more positive without having to think about it.

To finish up, over the page is my gratitude action plan. It includes actions that help me to find gratitude in the small things, and that give me a reality check any time I feel myself falling into the 'more' trap. Gratitude is a powerful thing. It can seriously change your whole mindset. I won't lie, you have to actually make an effort, but I promise you it's worth it. When you give it a red-hot go, I'm sure you'll soon start to reap the benefits every day, just as I have.

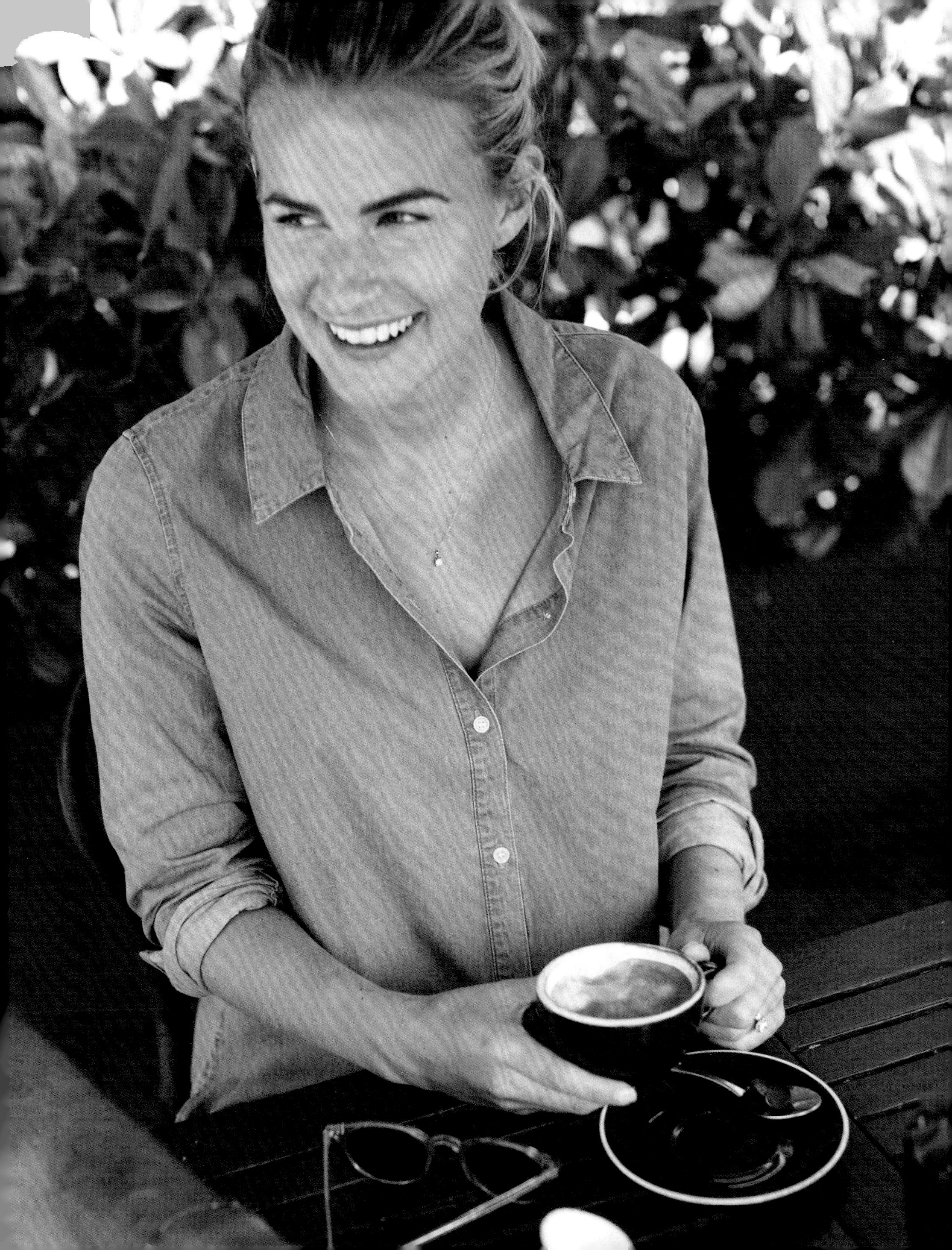

THE GRATITUDE ACTION PLAN

* Think about all the things you DO have, rather than what you don't. It could be your family, your friends, your pets, your intelligence, your sense of humour, a roof over your head—pretty much anything. You're allowed to be grateful for these things.

* Don't just think a compliment. VOICE IT. I've started doing this, and it's amazing how much joy it brings both me and the person I'm complimenting. I love it! Think of a time you got a compliment from a stranger. It made you feel pretty good, am I right? I'll never forget the time an old lady at the supermarket told me I looked 'as cool as a cucumber' in my outfit. It completely turned my day around. A good little challenge is to spend a day voicing every positive thought you have about others. It might feel unusual, but that's just a sign we should do it more.

* Put your phone away when you're with other people. You'll be better placed to experience their company fully. It shows them you are present, and that you're appreciating and listening to them. Ever been out for dinner and someone has whipped out their phone to start scrolling through their social media notifications? It's super rude, and it basically says, 'I think this post from this person who I don't even know is more interesting and important than you are right now.'

* Keep a gratitude journal. There are so many out there to buy that already have everything handily set out for you—just do an internet search for 'gratitude journal', and you'll see what I mean. You can also just use a good old notepad and pen, or even keep notes on your phone! Every evening, write down three things that you are grateful for and three things that made you smile that day.

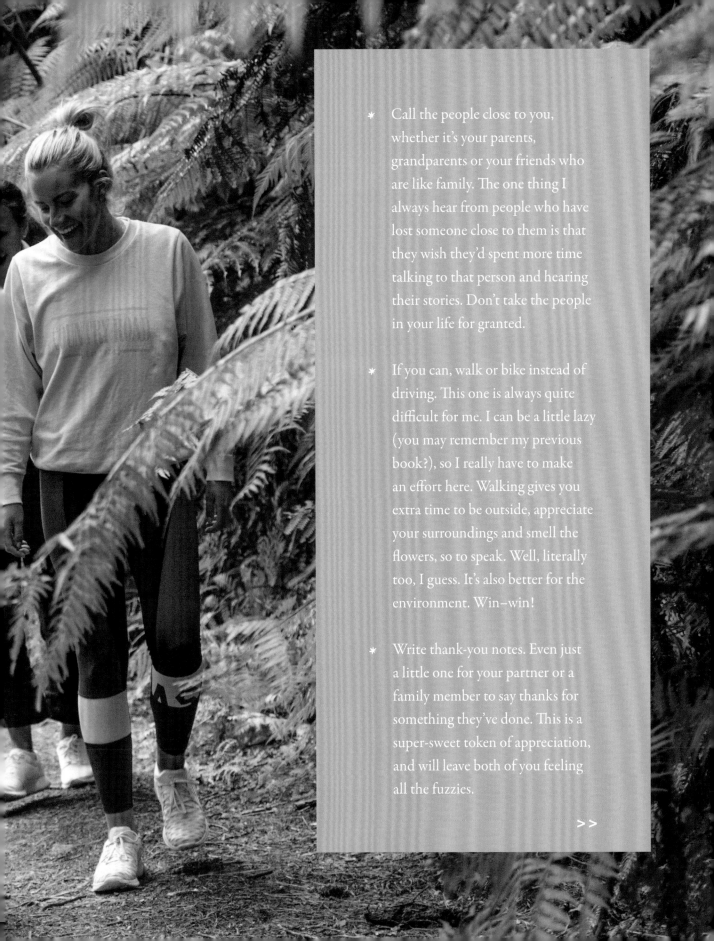

* Call the people close to you, whether it's your parents, grandparents or your friends who are like family. The one thing I always hear from people who have lost someone close to them is that they wish they'd spent more time talking to that person and hearing their stories. Don't take the people in your life for granted.

* If you can, walk or bike instead of driving. This one is always quite difficult for me. I can be a little lazy (you may remember my previous book?), so I really have to make an effort here. Walking gives you extra time to be outside, appreciate your surroundings and smell the flowers, so to speak. Well, literally too, I guess. It's also better for the environment. Win–win!

* Write thank-you notes. Even just a little one for your partner or a family member to say thanks for something they've done. This is a super-sweet token of appreciation, and will leave both of you feeling all the fuzzies.

> >

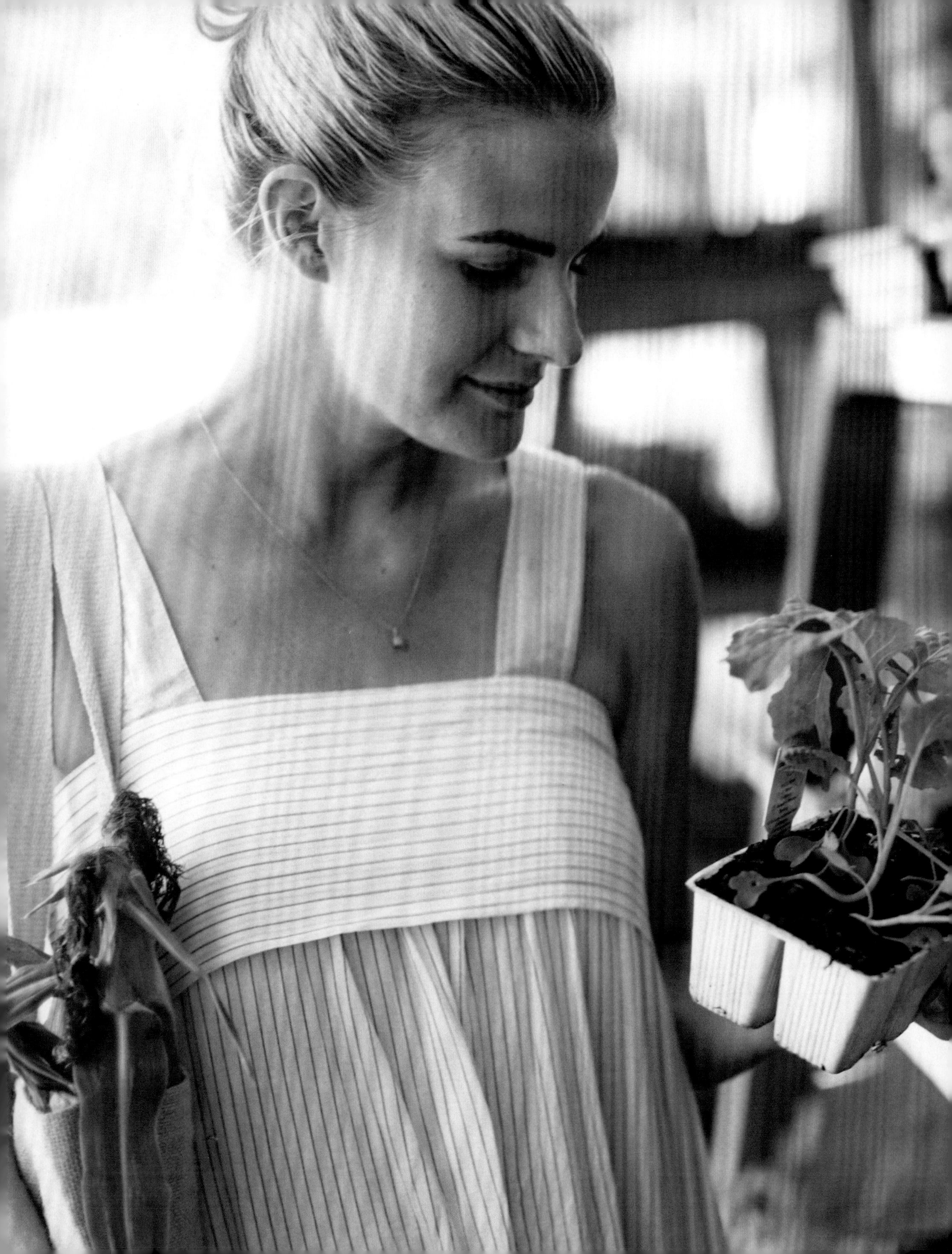

* Pay it forward. When someone does something nice for you, do something nice for someone else. Such a simple but powerful idea. Imagine if everyone in the world did this!

* Be OK with apologising. Saying sorry is actually a sign of strength, not of weakness. I've learnt that being right all the time doesn't mean much if you have hurt someone in the process.

* Help people out. I personally think that, to lead a happy and fulfilled life, you need purpose, and purpose comes from helping other people. We are all connected, and we need to look after each other. Plus, there's nothing wrong with admitting that helping people also makes you feel good. It's a win–win! There are lots of ways you can help someone out. Volunteer for a charity, help a neighbour with their garden, or just be there for your friends when they're having a hard time. Big or small, it all counts.

* Leave positive reviews. Had a good experience in a restaurant? A noticeably friendlier-than-average customer service rep? Let people know! Tell their manager or leave a review online. If you've ever worked in customer service or hospo, you'll know it can be hard yakka with little to no thanks, so when someone takes time out of their day to acknowledge you've done a good job it is certainly appreciated. It doesn't fall on deaf ears.

* Appreciate your food's journey. This one is a suggestion from my husband, Art, bless him. Whenever Art eats one of his favourite meals (steak and veggies), he takes a moment to send respect to the animal that gave their life so he could eat, and he thinks about the farms and the hard work that went into growing and harvesting the vegetables he's eating. I really like this one!

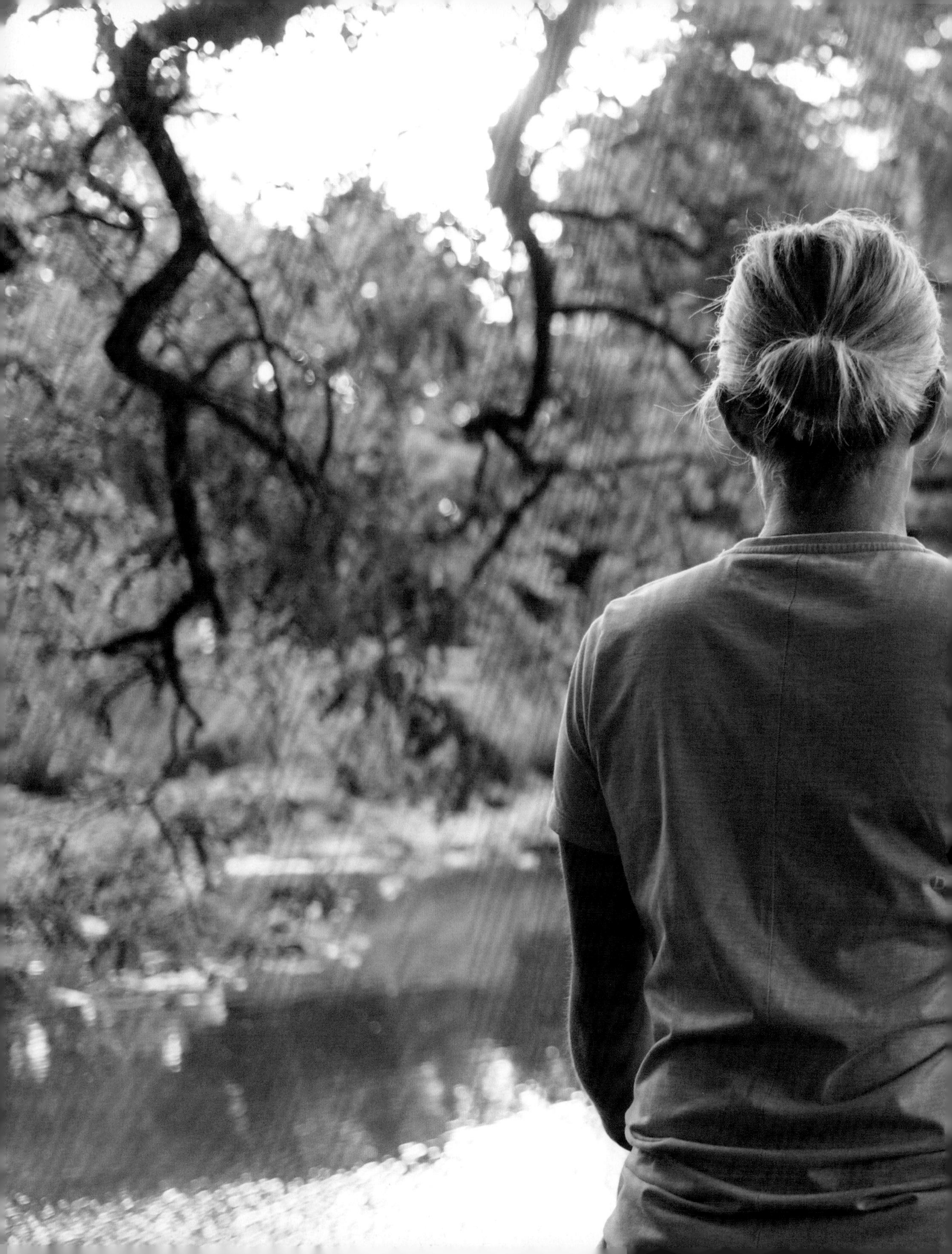

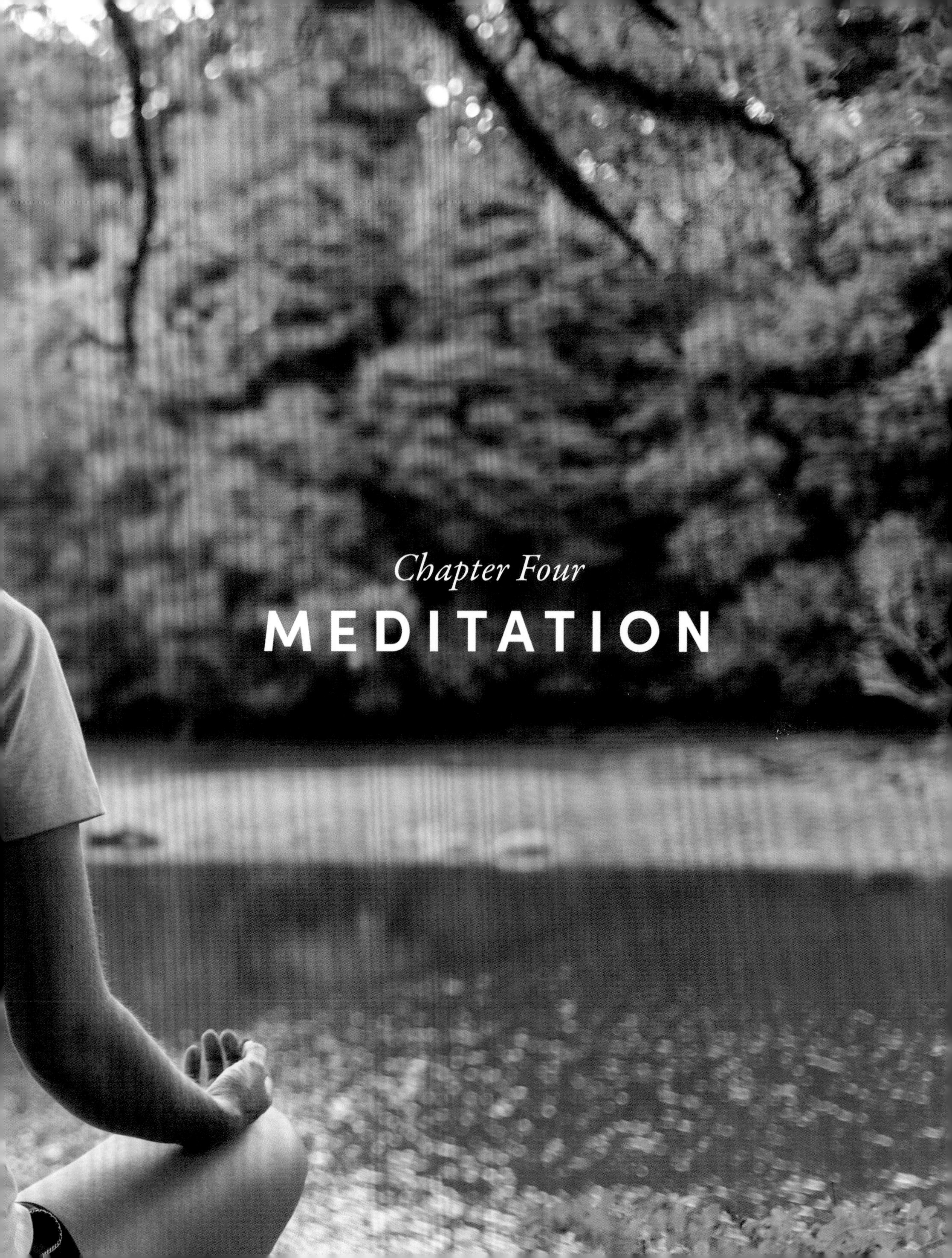

Chapter Four

MEDITATION

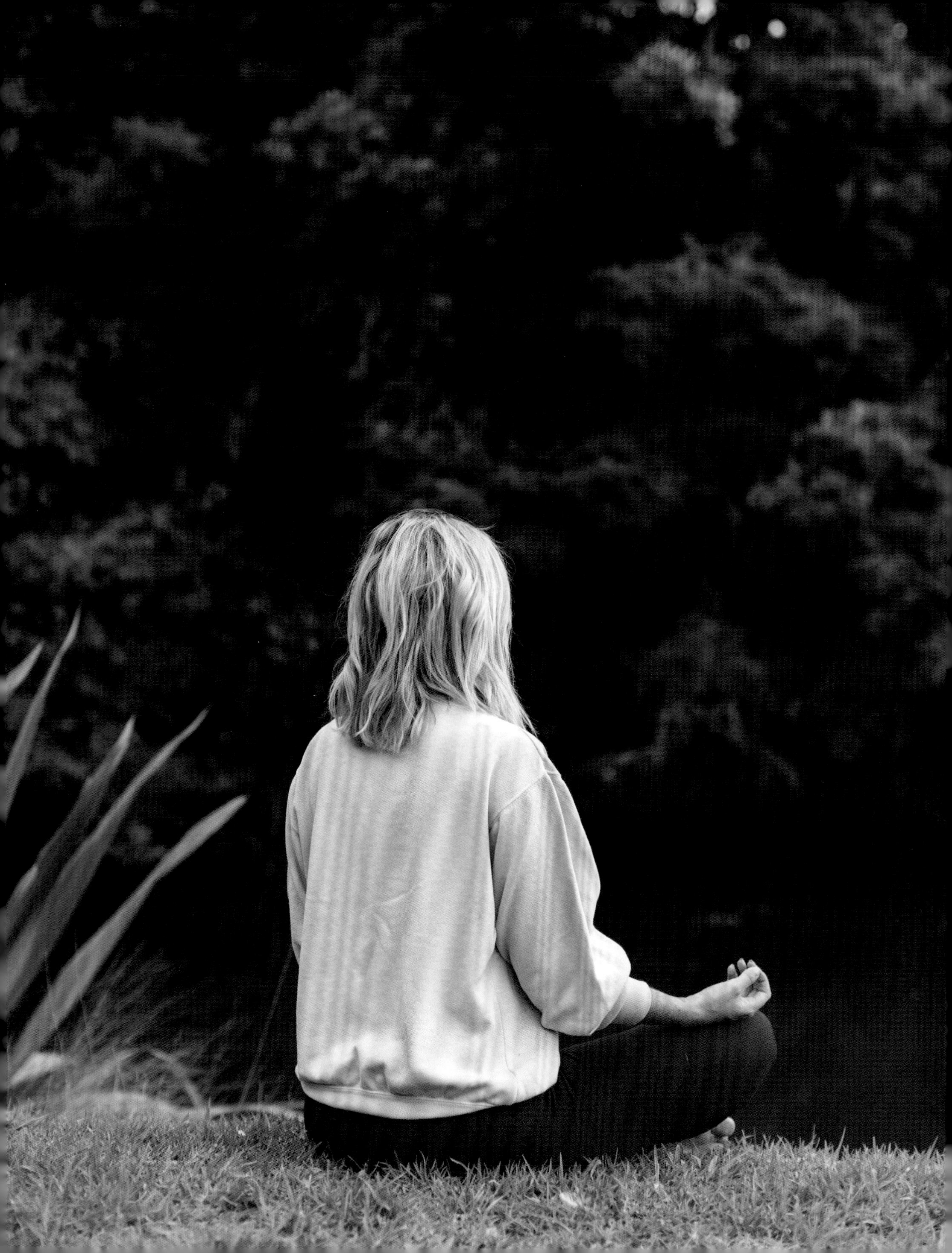

When someone says the word 'meditation' to you, what do you think of? Be honest. Do you picture someone sitting on a mountaintop somewhere idyllic, their legs crossed and both forefingers and thumbs curled into little circles while their hands rest on their knees and they're humming 'Ommmmmm'? They're probably plonked in the same sort of setting as all those people who do tree poses on Instagram, right?

You might have even given meditation a go once or twice . . . and decided it's not really your jam. Lots of people make it look like it's the easiest thing in the world, posting photos online of themselves being all peaceful and Zen, but in real life a lot of people can find meditation (or even just *trying* to meditate) has the opposite effect. It just makes them more stressed because they can't relax! Then they get frustrated at themselves because they can't relax, and then eventually they give up.

I'm not going to pretend that this wasn't me the first few times I tried meditating. I battled, and I wasn't actually sure I was even doing it. But I can tell you I'm really pleased I came back to it, and stuck to it, because it's ended up being a huge help to me. It's now firmly a part of my life.

One of the main things I had to work out was that meditation has nothing to do with how you look on the outside and everything to do with what's going on within, so all those social media posts are really just a big old distraction. (Anyone picking up on a theme here?) So, if you're one of the many, many people out there who think meditation is just not your bag and it's only for hippies, I'm here to ask you to open your mind just a tiny bit. Just give it one more try. (I can tell you're a bit curious, or you wouldn't have picked up this book—and you certainly wouldn't have made it this far.)

Meditation's definitely not for everyone, but you have to try something properly before you decide you don't like it, right? If, once you've given meditation a good go, you still absolutely hate it and never want to do it again, that's totally fine. There are a heap of other ways to calm your mind and body, like practising gratitude, mindfulness or even a spot of yoga perhaps. It's all about finding what works best for you.

WHAT EVEN IS MEDITATION?

Meditation is a bit of a tricky one to come right out and define because, well . . . it's meditation. It's not really one set thing. There are SO many different ways that so many different people meditate all over the world. The only thing you can really do is give a few different types of meditation a go, and then work out what meditation is for *you*.

To me, meditation is a practice that gives me time to completely relax my body and my mind, while also descrambling my brain. It's a way for me to check in with how I'm feeling both physically and spiritually. I like to think of it as a big mental hug.

These days, lots of us (well, most of my generation, at least) never give our brain a moment to be still or unoccupied. Most of us feel uncomfortable when our brain is still. We *hate* being bored or having nothing to do—hence why we pick up our phones when we're doing nothing or are waiting for food or feel uncomfortable sitting alone. And, if we're not on our phones, we'll watch

To me, meditation is a practice that gives me time to completely relax my body and my mind, while also descrambling my brain. It's a way for me to check in with how I'm feeling both physically and spiritually. I like to think of it as a big mental hug.

a show. Then, off we go to bed . . . and we just lie there, with our brain going a hundred miles a minute and totally unable to turn our thoughts off.

I believe this is because too many of us don't give our brain time during the day to rest. We don't give it a moment that's unstimulated. So, it's only once the day is done and the lights are off that our brain finally has a chance to catch up on everything that's happened. It ends up trying to process things right when we're trying to sleep. Sound familiar?

Meditation is, in part, about giving your brain the downtime it needs during the day so your thoughts don't keep you awake at night. It's about finding comfort in being still, and accepting and observing your own thoughts and emotions without letting them consume you.

MEDITATION AND ME

I always knew *about* meditation, but for a long time I didn't really know exactly *what* it was. I didn't understand the relevance of it to a non-spiritual person like myself. (This was pre-spiritual me, obviously.) I actually can't remember exactly when I first tried meditation, but I do remember that I found it difficult. I thought it was solely about 'clearing' the mind, so I found it really frustrating when I couldn't do that. It was like the more I tried to *not* think, the more my brain went crazy and started thinking about everything under the sun.

So I gave up on it for a while, thinking it wasn't for me.

Then, in 2018, our friends Nick and Danica, who run a mindfulness business called Joyful, invited Art and me to go with them on a happiness retreat in Byron Bay that they were organising. I had no idea what to expect, but I wanted to go into it with an open mind. In total, there were ten of us on the retreat. We all came from completely different backgrounds and had completely different personalities, but we were connected by our desire to learn more about mindfulness and the effect it could possibly have on our lives.

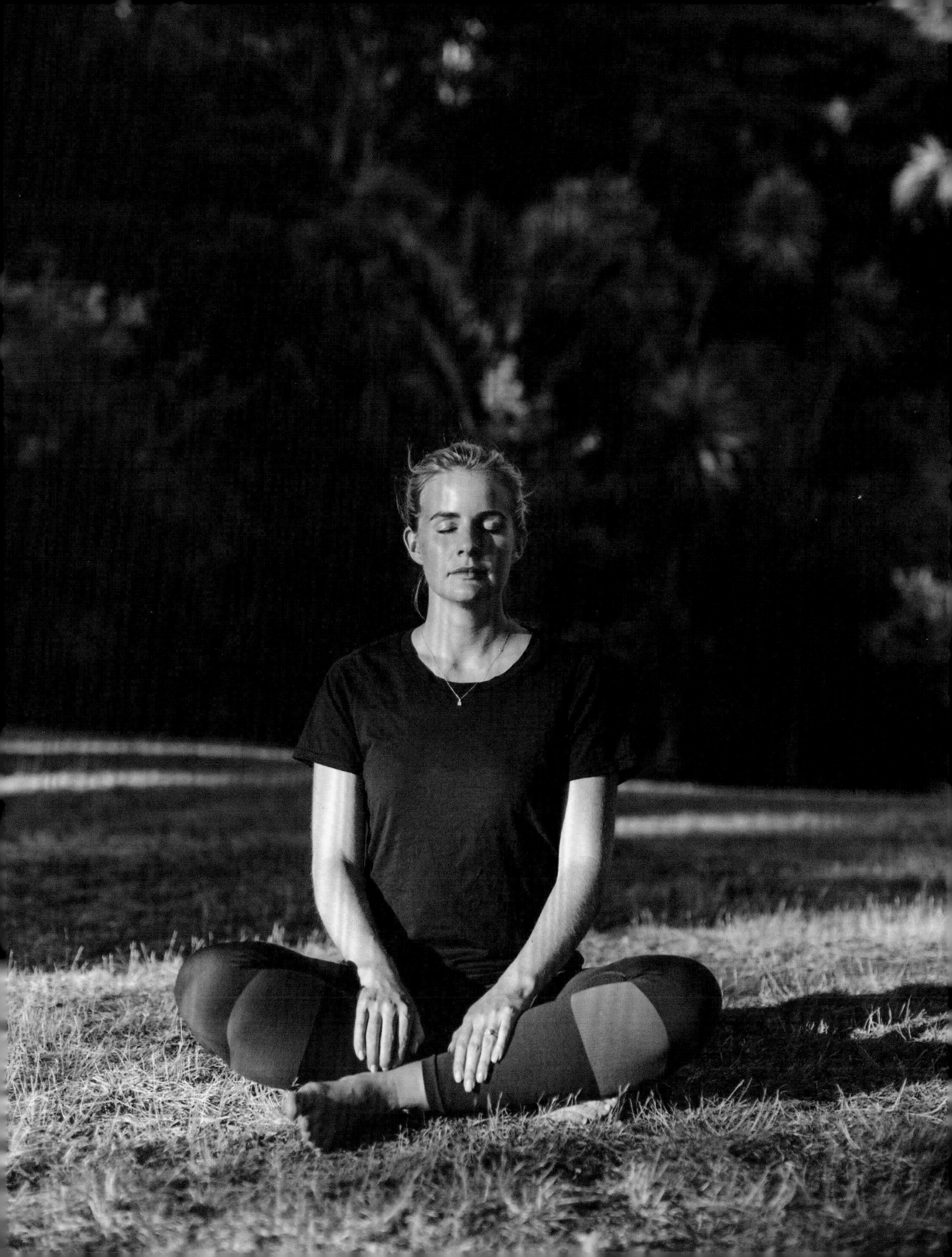

These days, I make meditation one of my main priorities for my health, simply because I've seen so many improvements since I started.

Some of us were further along the mindfulness journey than others—I was just starting out, so it was great to learn from more seasoned spiritual peeps. I tell you, I learnt so much on that retreat! I'll cherish my time there forever. As well as finally teaching me about what meditation really is, Nick and Danica encouraged me to let go of any expectations I had about what meditation 'should' be. Among other things, that trip really opened my eyes to my spiritual side—something that I hadn't actually realised I had.

After the retreat, I continued to learn more about meditation. I began to understand that it's not about being perfect at a certain practice. Instead, it's about taking time to be still, to reduce stress, to separate yourself from your thoughts, and to just get involved in your spiritual side. Explore it a bit! Once I discovered this view on what meditation is, I truly began to experience the benefits.

Now, with the benefit of hindsight, I can see that one of the reasons I used to struggle so much with meditation was because I was putting too much pressure on the end result. I have a habit of having really high expectations of myself, then getting frustrated and giving up on things if I'm not instantly good at them. Which is quite funny, because I'm not instantly good at most things. In fact, I can't even think of one thing I've been instantly good at. Oh, wait. Maybe golf? I have been told I'm a natural . . . (May as well fit in a horn-toot there.)

THE BENEFITS OF MEDITATION

Lots of people who practise meditation regularly will happily tell you all about what a good effect it's had on their mental and physical well-being—and I'm actually one of them.

These days, I make meditation one of my main priorities for my health, simply because I've seen so many improvements since I started. I know that sticking to it is absolutely worth it. Some of these personal benefits include the following.

* **My road rage has gone.** OK, this is quite embarrassing for me to admit, but I used to suffer from extreme road rage. I always considered myself quite a calm person, but when I was driving it was as if my built-up aggression and stress all came out. I would yell, swear, flip the bird—you name it! It would actually really scare poor Art. I didn't think it was an issue, until I realised a few months after starting meditation that my road rage had almost completely disappeared. To me, this is a brilliant example of how meditation has helped to prevent my emotions consuming me. I can deal with stress much more easily, as I'm able to separate myself from my emotions.

* **I find it much easier to practise forgiveness.** Ever heard that popular saying that holding on to anger is like drinking poison and expecting the other person to die? Better to let go of negative thoughts and feelings, and I think meditation has helped me to do that.

* **I can concentrate for sustained periods of time.** This is a huge one for me. I have always had a lot of trouble concentrating on just one thing for an extended period of time, as my mind tends to be all over the place. My attention span used to be lacking a tad, but has now significantly improved (which significantly helped with writing this book, actually!).

And, you know what else? Meditation has had a really positive impact on my self-esteem. I think this is because it's helped me to realise that my thoughts

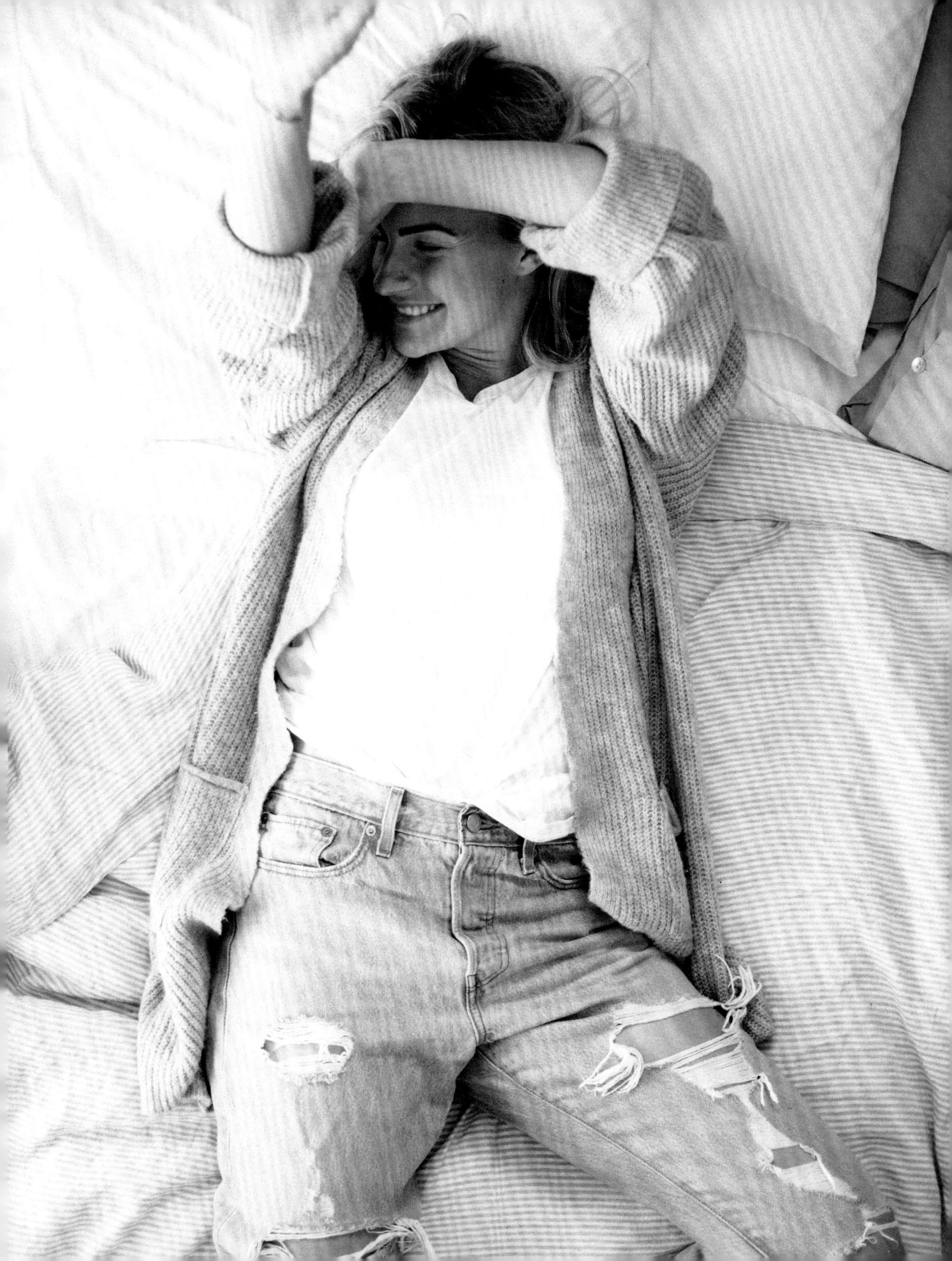

It has also helped me to realise that life doesn't just stop with me. It's also about caring for others and giving to them. Which, in turn, gives back to you!

don't define me. My thoughts aren't *me*, if you catch my drift. They're just things that pop into my head. So, if I have negative or self-doubty thoughts, I don't have to listen to them. I can just let them pass on by, safe in the knowledge that they're simply thoughts. Nothing more. This is something that we all need to remember, as those negative thoughts can certainly be a bit loud sometimes.

In this way, all the meditation I've done has helped me to realise that I am enough. I've accepted myself, and all my strengths and weaknesses. It has also helped me to realise that life doesn't just stop with me. It's also about caring for others and giving to them. Which, in turn, gives back to you! In a spiritual way, I mean—not material!

But you don't just have to listen to me. There's also been a fair bit of research into the positive effects meditation can have. In one paper, published in 2019 in the *Journal of Occupational Health Psychology*, the researchers suggested that short guided mindfulness meditations practised multiple times a week could improve well-being and work stress with, in their words, 'potentially lasting effects'. The paper, titled 'Mindfulness on-the-go: Effects of a mindfulness meditation app on work stress and well-being', documented the effects of meditation on the psychological well-being, work stress and blood pressure of 238 healthy UK employees. For the trial, one group of participants was instructed to meditate once a day using a mindfulness app, while the control group didn't do any meditation. All of the participants filled in questionnaires before the trial began, then again four months later. The meditators reported a significant increase in psychological well-being and a significant decrease in anxiety and stress levels. Cool, huh?

One huge ongoing study has even shown that meditation can literally change your brain! The ReSource project (resource-project.org) is one of the longest and most comprehensive studies on the effects of meditation-based mental training to date. In 2018, Tania Singer, one of the researchers, published an essay titled 'What Type of Meditation Is Best for You?' in *Greater*

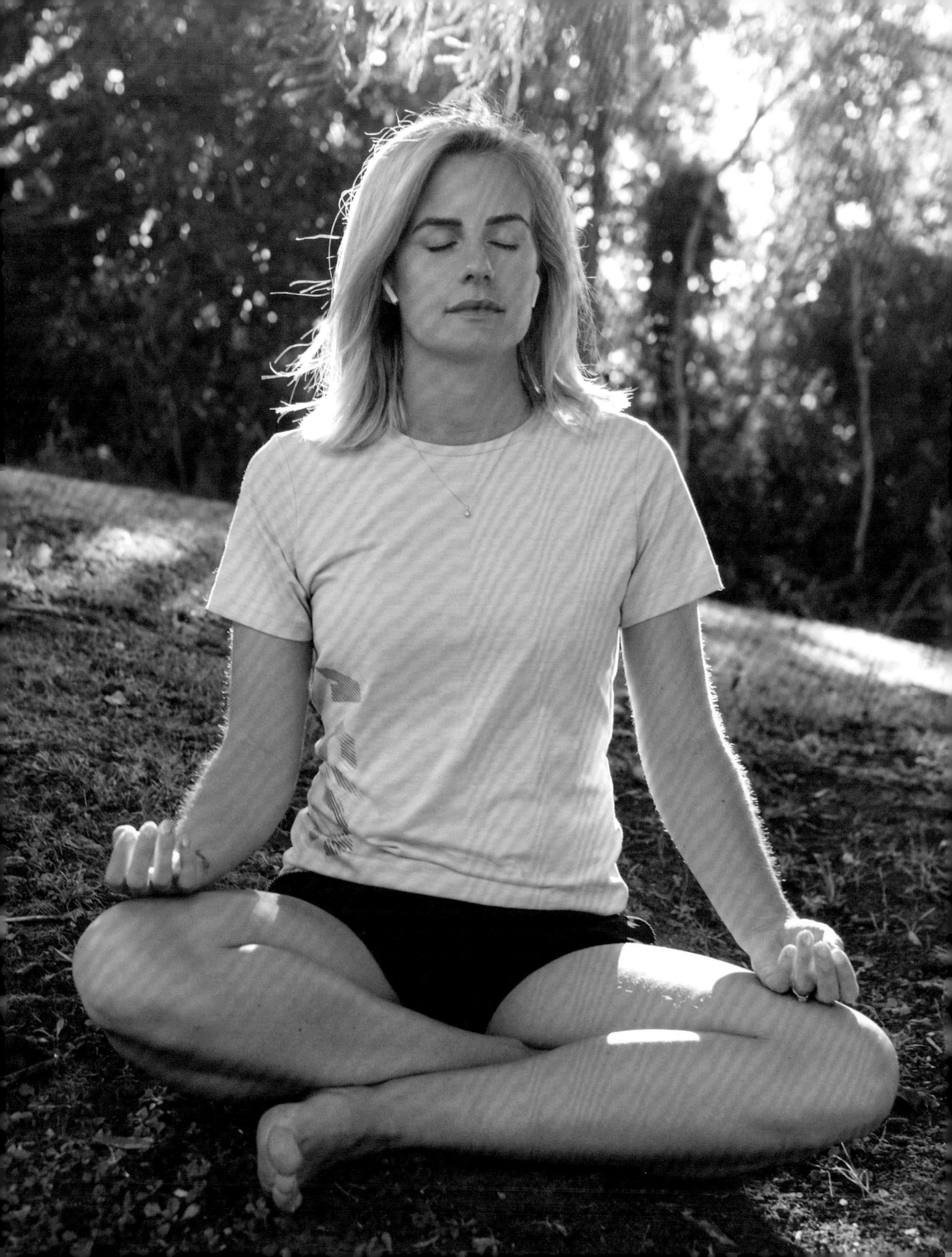

Good Magazine that documented some of the project's findings. In the essay, Singer described how researchers grouped mental-training practices into three different modules: presence (which included body-scan meditation), affect (which included loving-kindness meditation), and perspective. (More on these types of meditation on page 98.) They then asked over 300 German adults aged between 20 and 55 to attend a two-hour class every week, and practise for half an hour a day at home. The participants rotated through each module in a different order, and every three months were rigorously assessed with questionnaires, behavioural tests, hormonal markers and brain scans.

One of the most jaw-dropping findings was that certain types of practice changed the make-up of participants' brains in certain ways. As Singer explains, grey matter in the brain typically thins as people age—but, after three months of presence (mindfulness) training, participants showed a higher volume of grey matter in the areas of the brain related to attention, monitoring and higher-level awareness. After three months of affect training, by comparison, it was the areas involved in empathy and emotional regulation that became thicker. Pretty amazing stuff!

Put really simply, this study highlighted that the *type* of meditation you do actually matters, because different types of meditation result in different outcomes. So that's a great reason to try a whole heap of different styles of meditation and decide which ones are right for you.

GETTING STARTED

Now, I hope you're itching to have a go at meditating (or another go at it, as the case may be). Good for you!

You can meditate for as long as you like, but it's a good idea to start small— as in, do it for a couple of minutes a day—then work your way up to longer durations. You can also meditate anywhere you like. Just make sure to find a nice quiet space in which you won't be interrupted. (If you have a baby, maybe the perfect time is just when they fall asleep, so hopefully you can grab a couple of minutes to yourself!) And, when you do have a go, if you find yourself struggling to figure out the point, just remember this quote by Anonymous (that incredibly wise person *full* of pearlers): 'The goal of meditation isn't to control your thoughts. It's to stop letting them control you.' Let go of those thoughts, my friend.

To begin with, I would recommend using a guided meditation app. An app can really help when you're starting out, as it's actually bloody hard to jump straight into meditation without some guidance. So, grab your phone and some headphones, find a quiet place and get Zen. Here's a list of some apps you could try.

* **Headspace** (headspace.com) is one of the first meditation apps I ever heard of. This one is great, as it'll take you on a fully guided meditation journey for beginners. This app also makes it really easy to track your meditations, and you can even set reminders.

* **Calm** (calm.com) is so easy to use. The meditations are organised into really user-friendly categories, such as 'anxiety', 'sleep' and 'focus'. That means you don't really have to know anything about meditation to figure out where you want to start.

* **1 Giant Mind** (1giantmind.com) focuses on a specific meditation technique called 'Being', which the app founder created based on vedic meditation. Vedic meditation comes from India and has been practised for thousands of years. It uses a mantra, and is super simple to practise. I love this app, as it has a lot of support including things like tutorial videos.

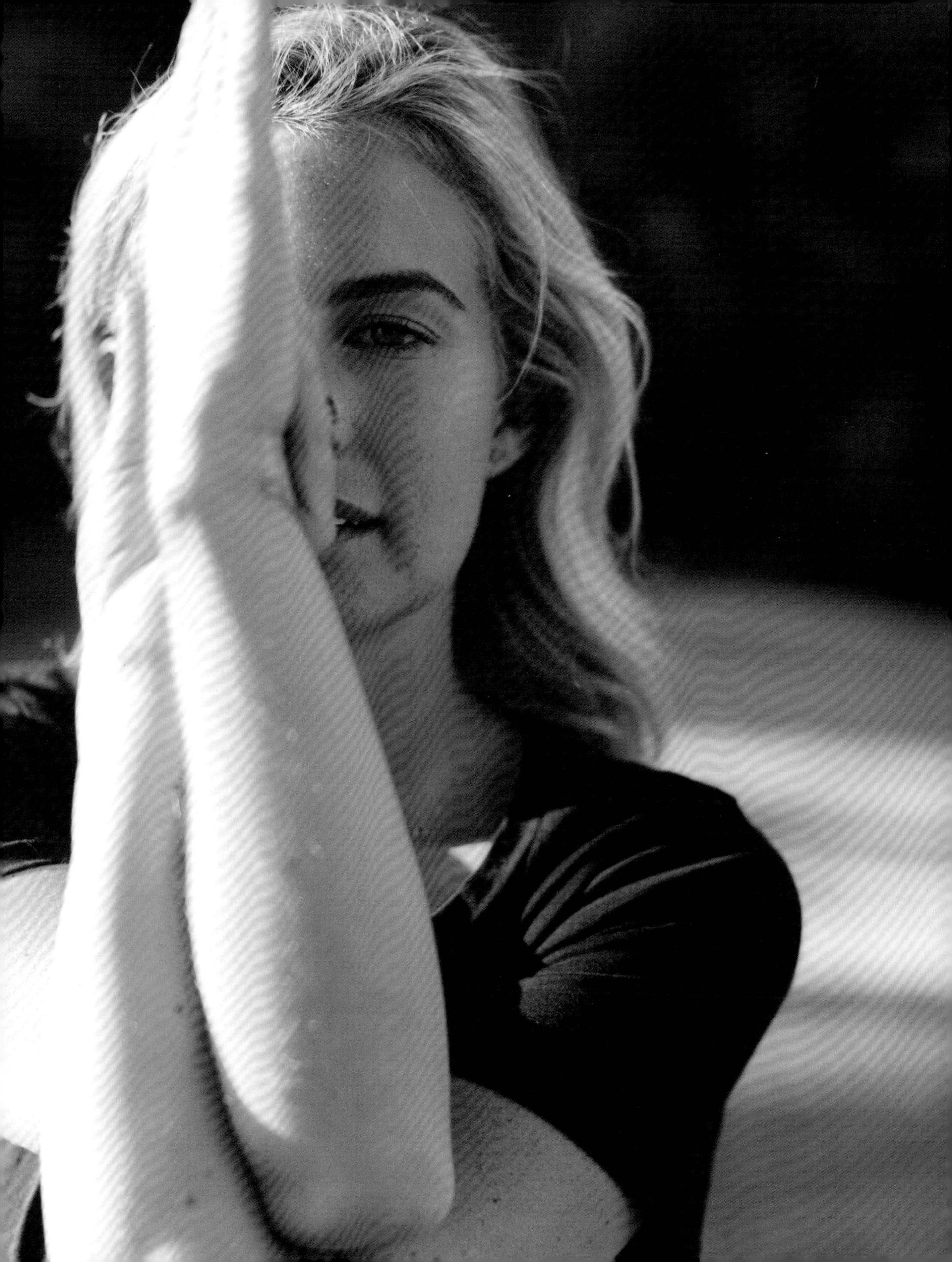

* **The Mindfulness App** (themindfulnessapp.com) is one
  I haven't used as much. There are, after all, only so many
  meditation apps one person can use at once! But this one is
  great, and even links in with quite a lot of other health apps,
  such as Lumosity (an app that helps you 'train your brain' with
  mental workouts).

* **Mindworks** (mindworks.org) is another really well set-out
  meditation app. It's super easy to use, and you can also do a
  fourteen-day free trial to decide whether you like it before
  committing to paying for it.

* **Insight Timer** (insighttimer.com) actually made *Time*
  magazine's list of the 50 best apps for 2016. Cool, right? It
  includes thousands of different meditations, and makes it
  really easy to search for the ones that work for you. I would
  recommend using Insight Timer after you've completed a
  guided meditation course or journey—there are SO many
  different styles of meditation that it can be a little overwhelming
  for a beginner unsure where to start.

Next thing: as I've already mentioned, there are lots of different ways to
meditate. I strongly advise you do a bit of your own research, and find out
about the different types of meditation that are out there. Find one or two
options that sound like they might suit you. To get you started, here are a few
of the different types of meditation that I've had a go at.

Loving-kindness meditation (mettā bhavana meditation)

This one is my personal favourite because it's just bloody lovely. The goal is to
basically turn your attitude towards everything into one of loving kindness.

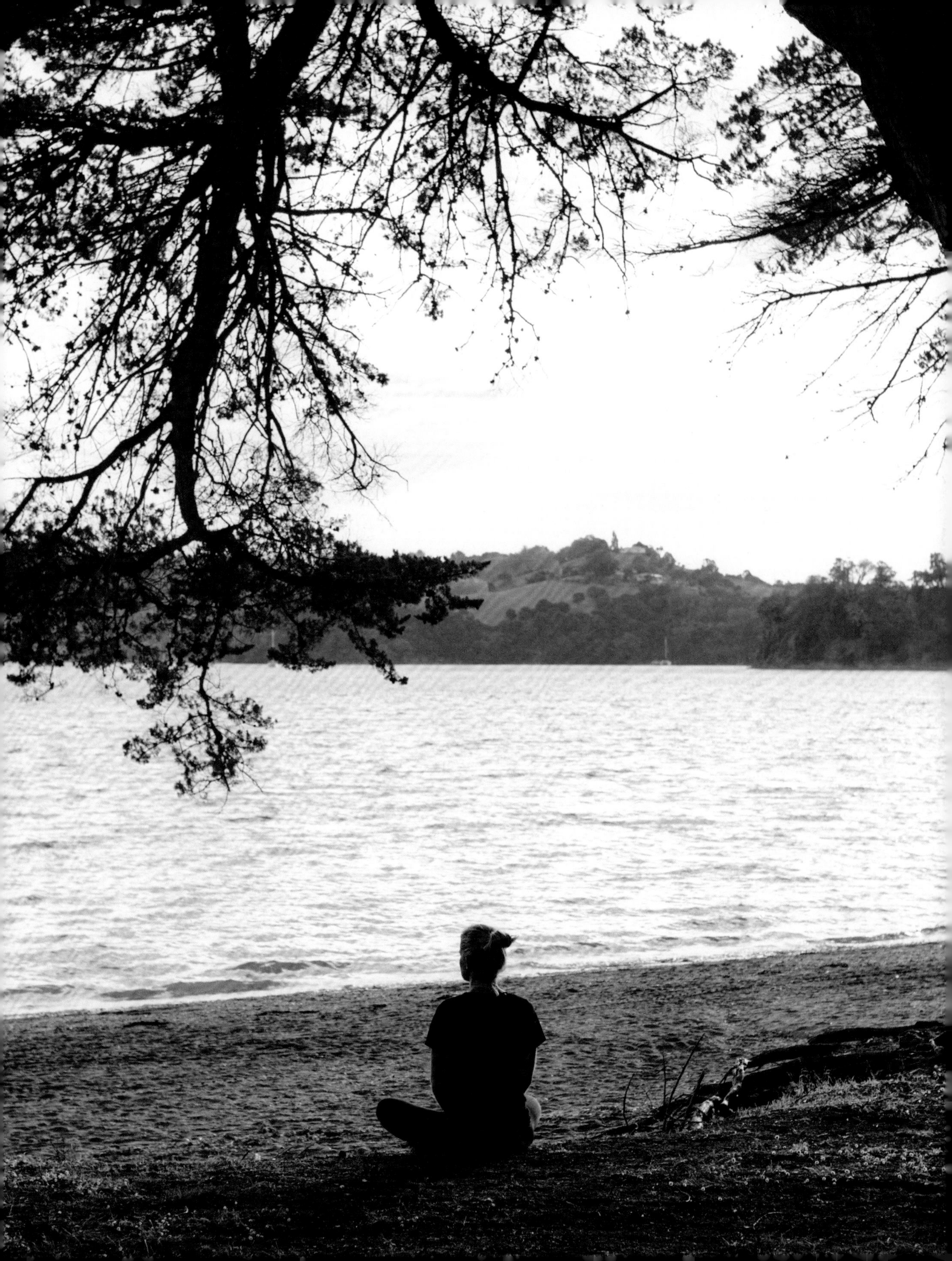

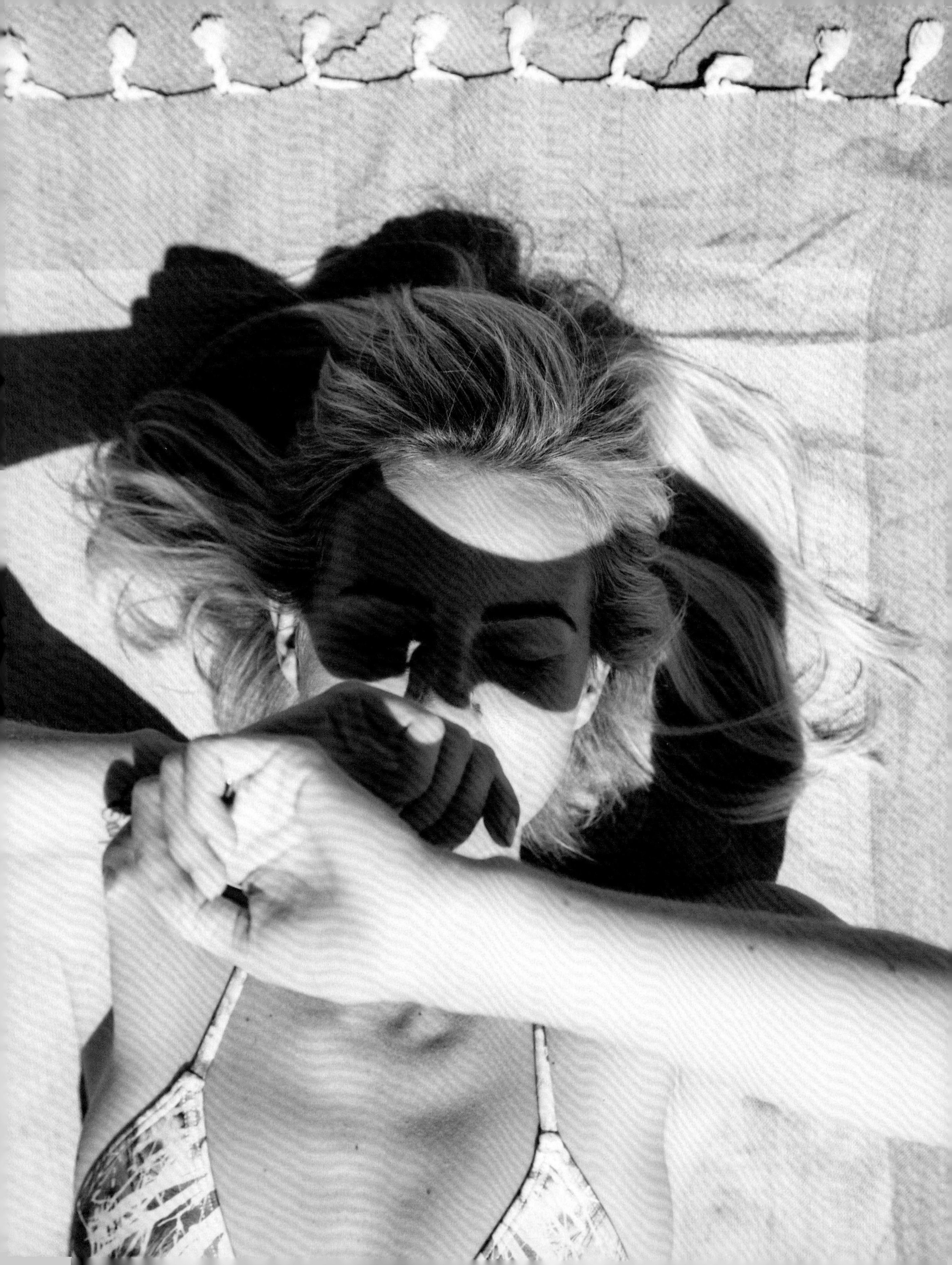

That can include anyone and anything—yourself, someone who you hold resentment for, friends, even the world.

The best way to have a go at this one is by using a guided meditation app such as Headspace, Insight Timer or Calm.

Progressive relaxation (body-scan meditation)

Progressive relaxation is a type of meditation that encourages people to scan their body for areas of tension or pain. The goal here is to notice any tension in the body, then actively focus on releasing it. Some people like to visualise a wave drifting over their body, while others visualise a light going through their body and 'scanning' it.

Progressive relaxation can help you to feel calm and relaxed. Some studies have also suggested that it may help with chronic pain, because it slowly and steadily relaxes the body. It's also a great form of meditation to help you sleep.

In order to try this one, I'd recommend starting with some guided body-scan meditations online. It's a little more difficult to do this one by yourself, as it can be tempting to rush it. (Well, that's what I do anyway.) Also, unless you already have a fantastic knowledge of the human body, I don't think it is quite as effective without guidance.

Zen meditation

Zen often forms part of a Buddhist practice. The goal is to slow down your breathing and focus on it, while calmly observing your thoughts without judgement. This is a common one in meditation apps like Headspace. It's also a great one to do on your own, as it's super simple, you can do it anywhere and it feels a little easier to practise unguided as the only thing you're focusing on is your breathing.

On the everyday level, Zen trains the mind to achieve calmness. It's also been suggested that people who meditate regularly are able to reflect with better focus and more creativity. According to the Mindworks app, improved physical health is another benefit, with people who practise Zen reporting lower blood pressure, reduced anxiety and stress, better immune systems and more restorative sleep.

Mantra meditation (vedic meditation)

For this meditation, once your breathing is centred and you feel grounded, you repeat a mantra either silently in your head or out loud. Your mantra can be anything, and you can also accompany it with visualising a goal in your mind. Traditionally, the mantras have been Hindu ones, but in more mainstream meditation they can be affirmations as well. It's good to keep your mantra short and easy to repeat. Maybe something like:

*   'I am confident.'

*   'I am love. I give love.'

*   'I am happy.'

The actual idea behind this form of meditation, according to the website doyouyoga.com, is to 'penetrate the depths of the unconscious mind and adjust the vibration of all aspects of your being'. So, ya know. Easy stuff.

A good app for this type of meditation is 1 Giant Mind.

I practise this sometimes when I have something I really want to focus on, but I don't do it that often as I personally prefer loving-kindness and body-scan meditations.

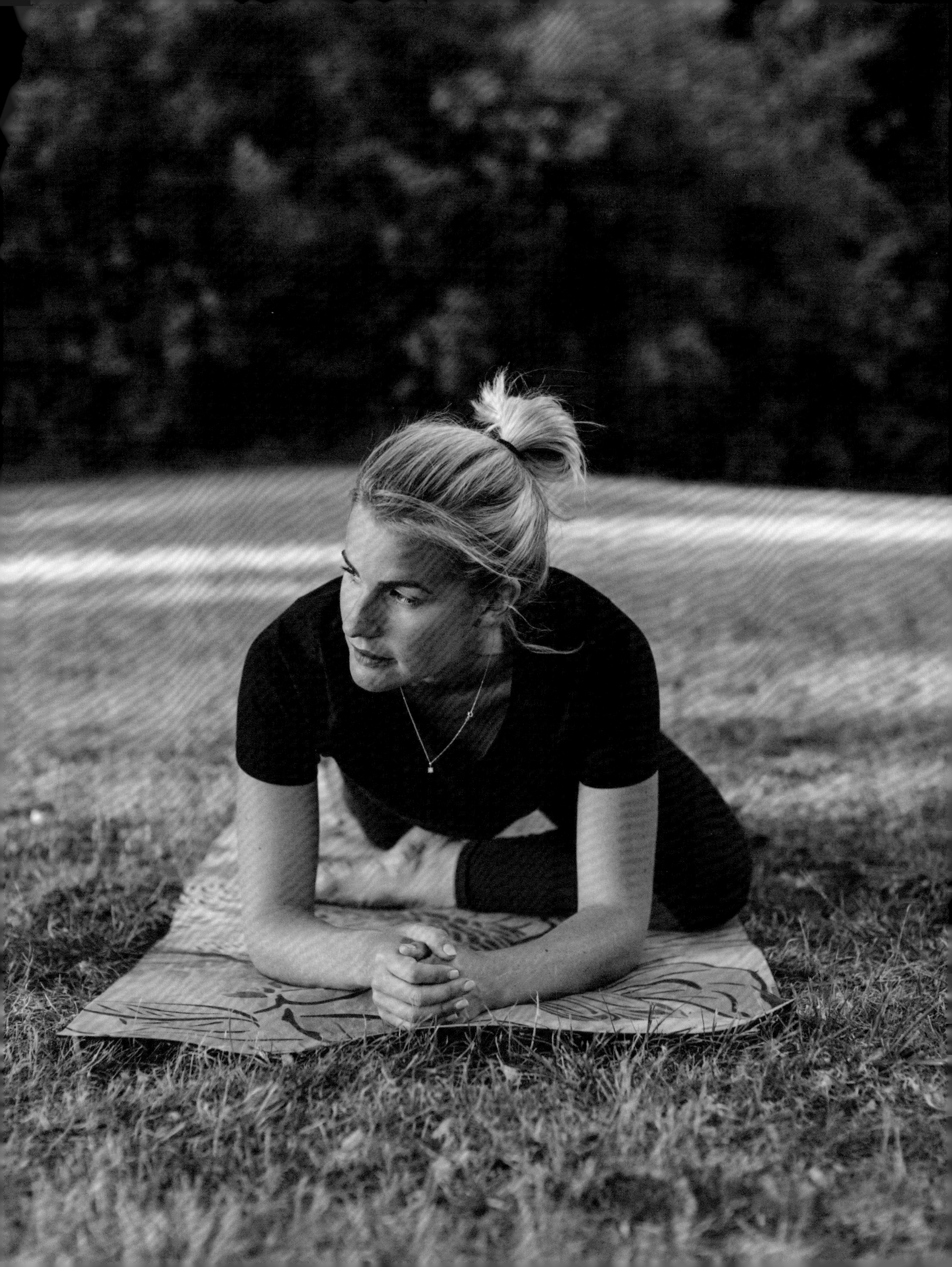

MY MEDITATION PRACTICE

In terms of my own meditation practice, I like to meditate for about
20 minutes a day, but some days I just can't be bothered (just being honest,
guys) so I only do a quick five. The trick is to just do whatever feels natural
at the time. I tend to practise loving-kindness meditation the most, as I find
it the most enjoyable. It just makes me feel all warm and fuzzy! I also really
enjoy the odd body-scan meditation. When I have time to meditate in the
morning, that's the time I prefer. Otherwise, I just do it whenever I can squeeze
it in during the day. I know that some people love to meditate just before bed
because it can help to calm the mind and drift you off to the land of nod.

Starting my day with some loving-kindness meditation in particular puts me
in such a good mood! Just one little meditation can turn my whole day around,
especially if I'm feeling a little grumpy or down to begin with. Most of the time
I do guided meditation with an app and headphones, but once or twice a week
I like to practise unguided—no phone, just me!—as it's good to not have to
always rely on an app.

All right, now you know what meditation is and have learnt about some of
the benefits it can have. It's time for you to leave the nest, grasshopper. Time to
put your newfound knowledge to the test! Because, at the end of the day, you
can read about meditation as much as you like, but nothing compares to just
giving it a go. A disclaimer, though: it's not a quick fix! It took me about two
months of solid practice to start to notice any changes, so it does take time.

Starting my day with some loving-kindness meditation in particular puts me in such a good mood! Just one little meditation can turn my whole day around.

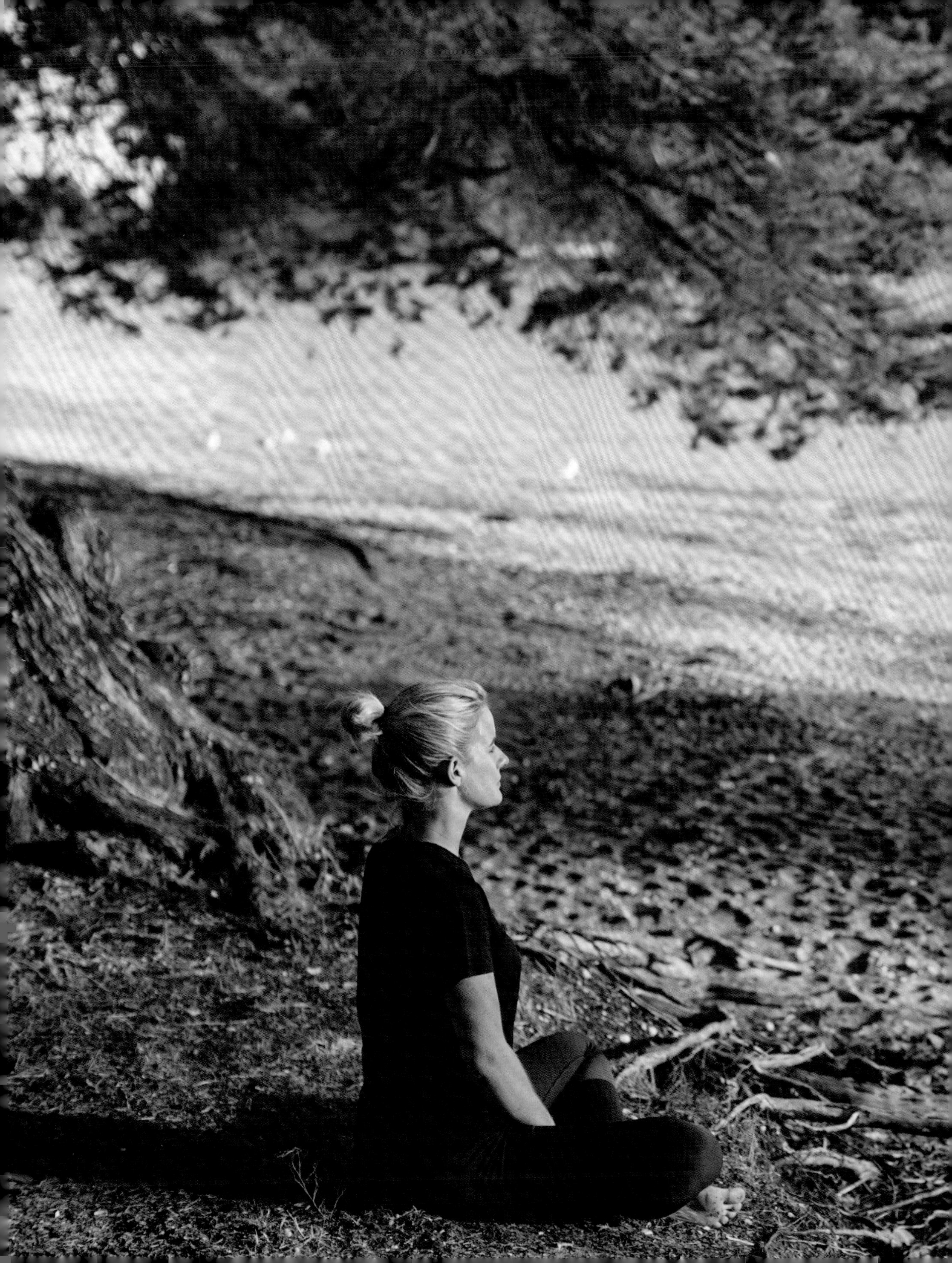

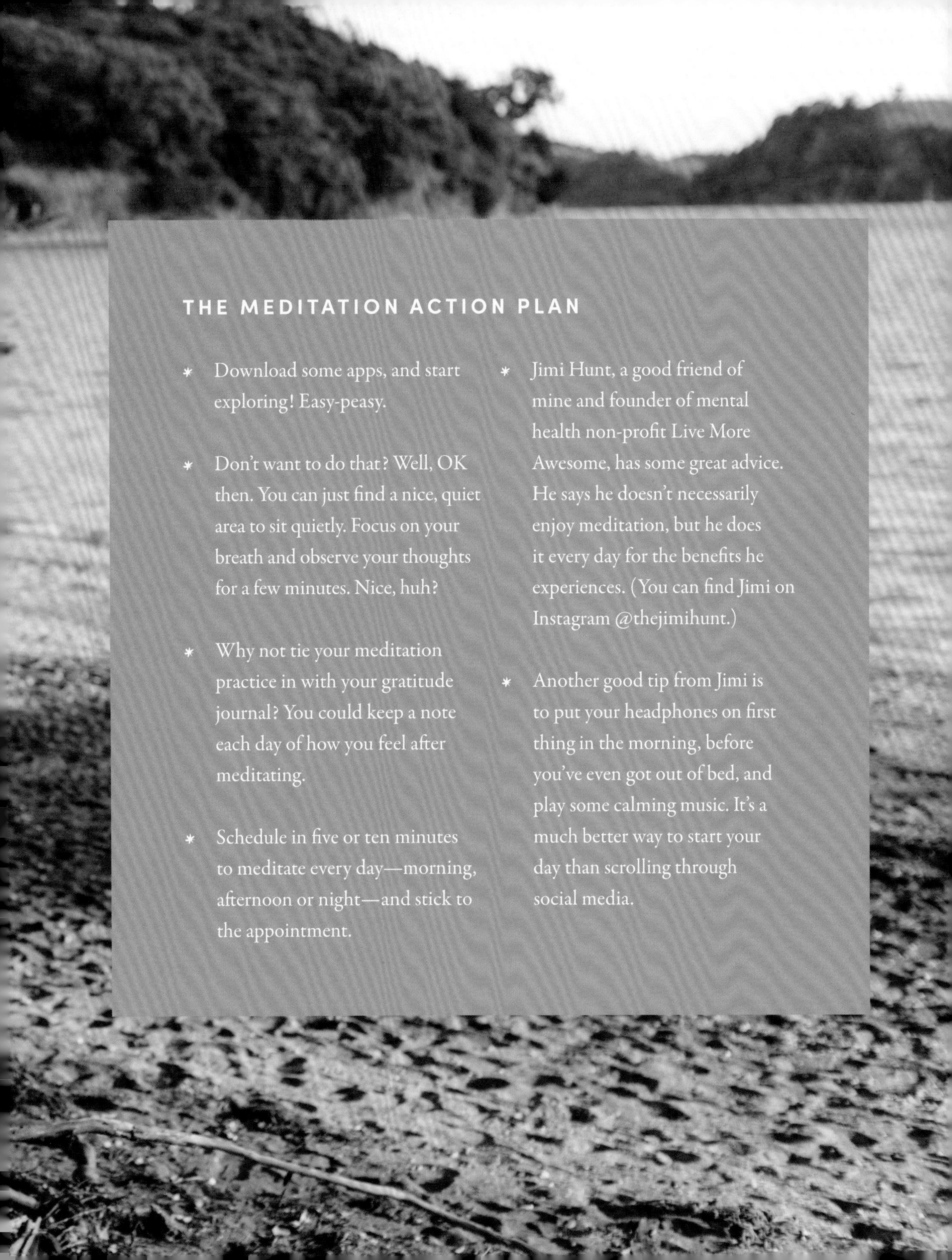

THE MEDITATION ACTION PLAN

* Download some apps, and start exploring! Easy-peasy.
* Don't want to do that? Well, OK then. You can just find a nice, quiet area to sit quietly. Focus on your breath and observe your thoughts for a few minutes. Nice, huh?
* Why not tie your meditation practice in with your gratitude journal? You could keep a note each day of how you feel after meditating.
* Schedule in five or ten minutes to meditate every day—morning, afternoon or night—and stick to the appointment.
* Jimi Hunt, a good friend of mine and founder of mental health non-profit Live More Awesome, has some great advice. He says he doesn't necessarily enjoy meditation, but he does it every day for the benefits he experiences. (You can find Jimi on Instagram @thejimihunt.)
* Another good tip from Jimi is to put your headphones on first thing in the morning, before you've even got out of bed, and play some calming music. It's a much better way to start your day than scrolling through social media.

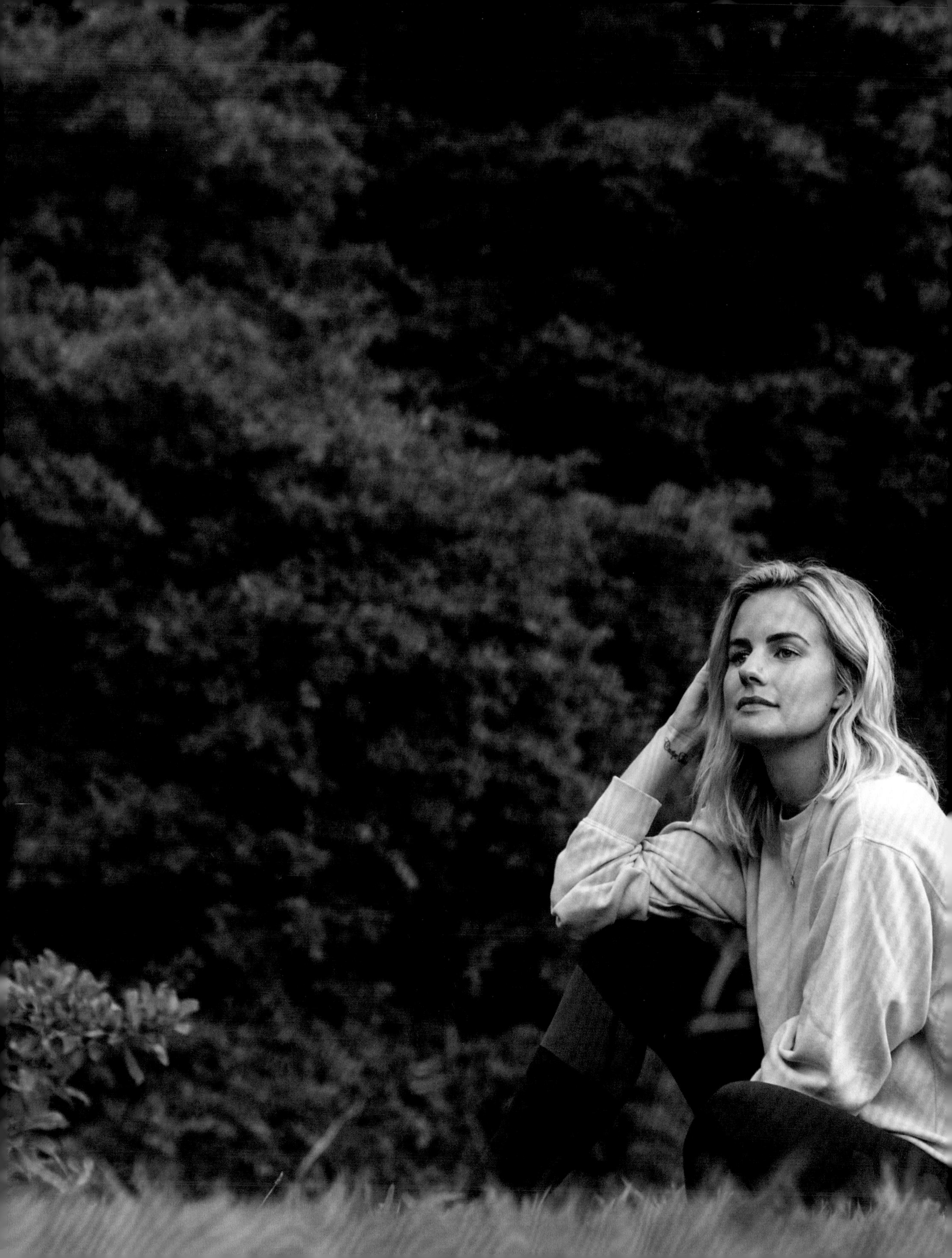

Chapter Five

MINDFULNESS

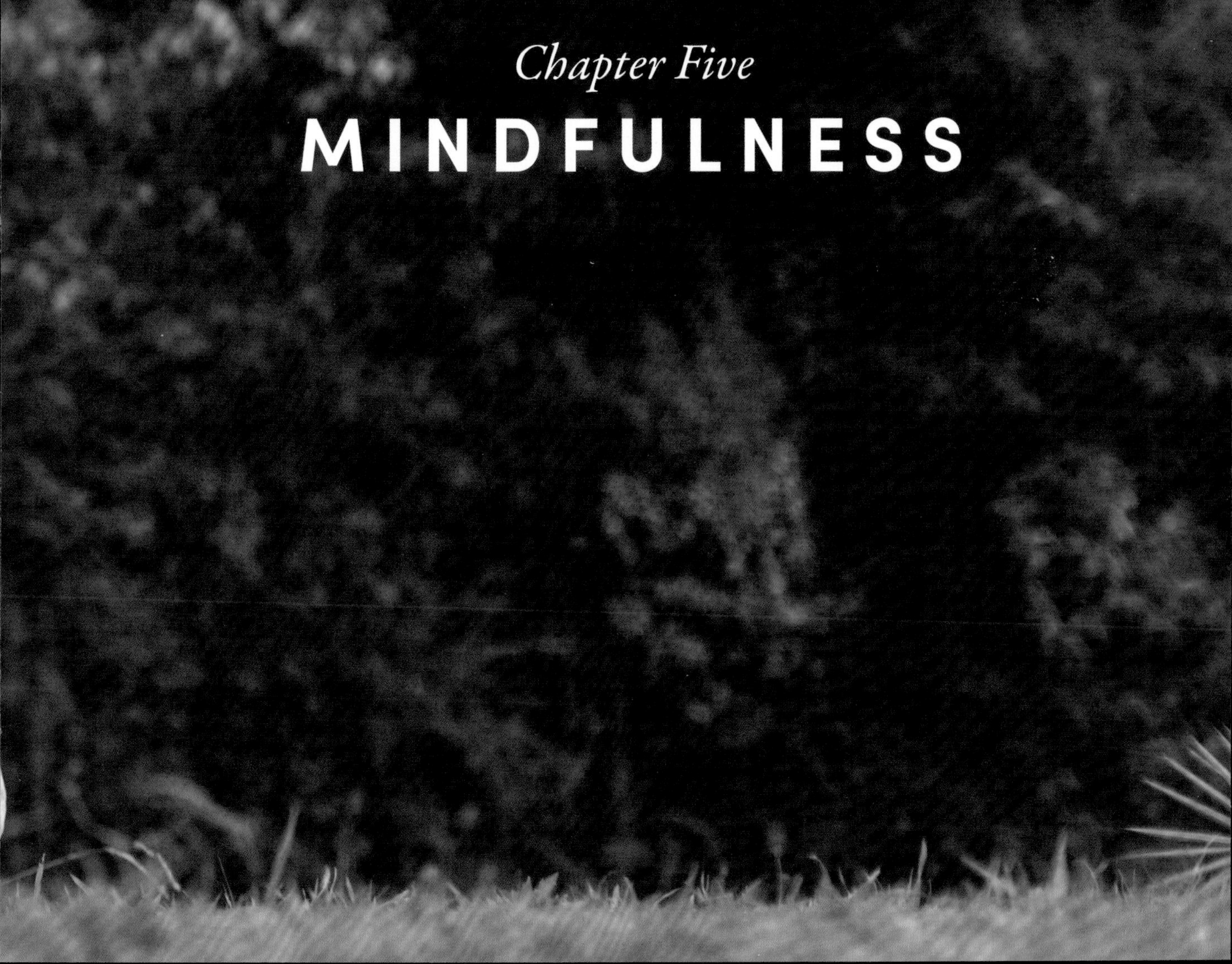

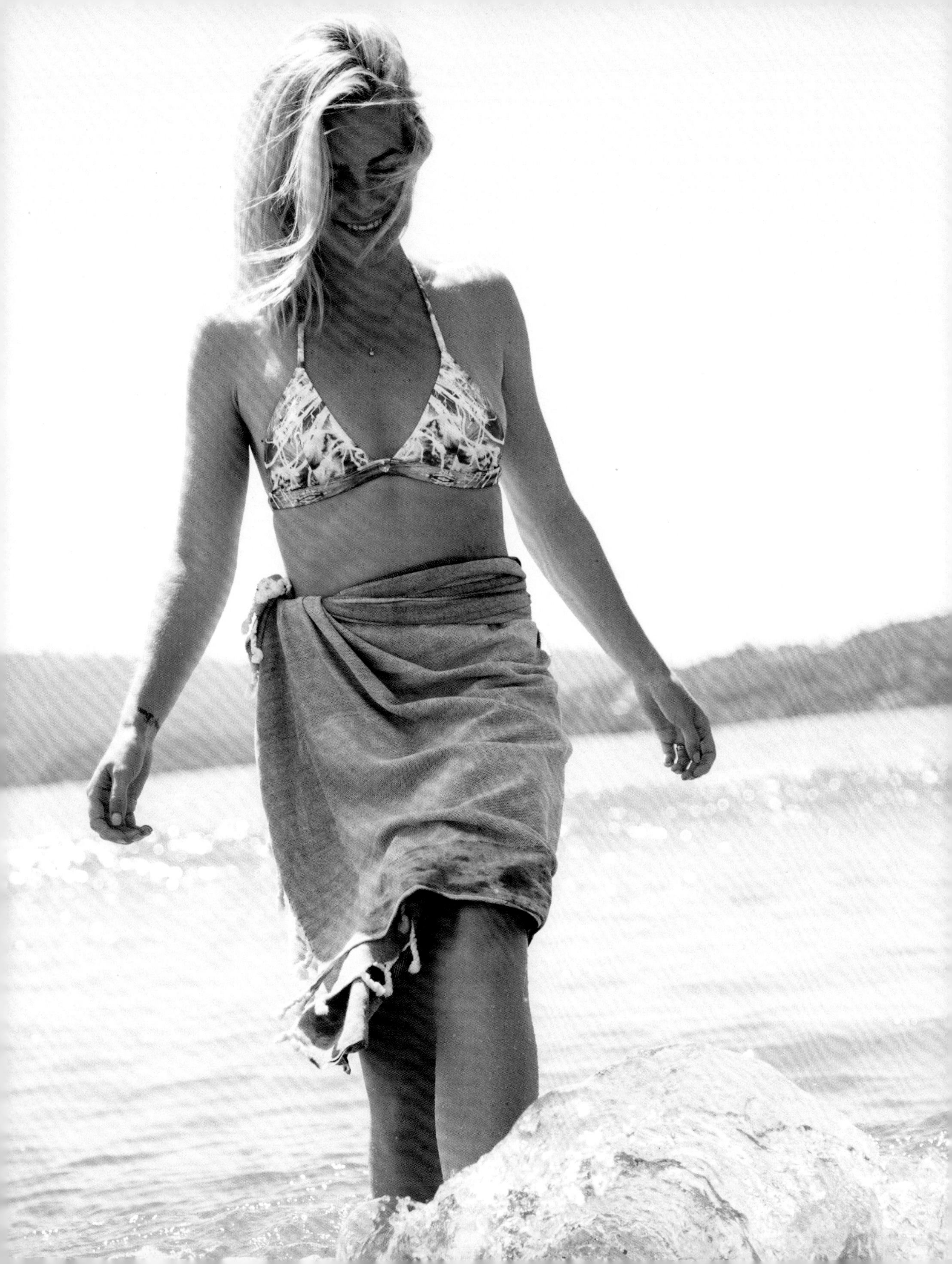

Meditation leads seamlessly (even if I do say so myself) into our next topic for discussion: mindfulness. Like gratitude and meditation, mindfulness has grown in popularity in recent years, and the three are actually all related. When you're practising gratitude or meditation, you're also practising mindfulness, even if you haven't realised it yet.

So, you're already a few steps ahead just by having read the last couple of chapters. Woop!

WHAT EVEN IS MINDFULNESS?

I have to admit, mindfulness is a pretty broad and confusing term. How does one define it? What does it mean to 'be mindful'? These are questions I have asked myself in the past, and these are the questions that hopefully I can clear up for you now.

Mindfulness essentially means being 'conscious' or 'aware', and acknowledging the present moment—including your thoughts, feelings, surroundings and so on. Are you reading this and thinking how trivial that sounds? That if we're present in person, then we're present in mind? Well, unfortunately that's not usually the case.

As I've already mentioned, we live in a world where, more often than not, our minds are going a million miles an hour, constantly analysing everything. Do you ever find yourself replaying a scenario from the past a hundred times over in your mind, thinking about all the ways it could have gone differently? Or maybe you spend a lot of time worrying about what's coming up in the future? Maybe you're anxious about a presentation at work, or a speech you have to give? Are you fretting so much about a big project that you're already telling yourself you're just never going to be able to find the time for it (even though you don't actually know that yet)? It might be something big and serious that's got you worrying, like bills (those pesky suckers) or climate change or terrorism. Or, it could be something as seemingly not-important as what you're going to have for dinner. It might be all of these things at the same time.

Often, we don't even realise that we're caught up in overthinking things, or ruminating. Our thoughts circle over and over and over the same territory. We can't stop our brain from thinking, even though if we took a step back we'd realise that obsessing about the same things repeatedly is going to do a big fat zero. A major part of mindfulness is learning how to recognise when you're caught in one of these thought loops in the first place.

Thought loops can cover every single topic, from big to small, from important to completely inconsequential, but in our heads every thought can start to feel as enormous and all-encompassing as every other thought. We think and think and think and think about EVERYTHING, so that we stop being able to tell the difference between what we actually *need* to think about and what we can stop thinking about because we've already spent enough time on it. It's scary when your mind starts to do this. It can feel like you're not even in the driver's seat any more. It can feel like the thoughts are controlling you, rather than the other way around.

The one thing that all of these sorts of thoughts do have in common is that they've actually got nothing to do with the present moment. And, most of the time, there's no relationship at all between how much we think about a

Often, we don't even realise that we're caught up in overthinking things, or ruminating. A major part of mindfulness is learning how to recognise when you're caught in one of these thought loops in the first place.

certain thing and the thing itself. All this ruminating pulls us away from the task at hand—being here, now, in the present—by distracting us with analysing the past and the future. We have no control over the past whatsoever, and the future has so many unknowns that it's just not worth stressing about.

And, of course, a mind full of thoughts that have taken over just contributes to that awful thing that all too many of us are all too familiar with: anxiety. This is sadly really common, and it's not a nice place to be.

MINDFULNESS (AND ANXIETY) AND ME

Lots of us feel anxious sometimes, and there are certain things that it's completely normal (and actually quite heathy) to feel anxious about. If you're about to do something you're nervous about or that you've never done before, it's completely unsurprising that you'd feel at least a wee bit anxious. In fact, it'd be more surprising if you didn't feel anxious.

Sometimes, feeling anxious can be a good thing. It's our brain's way of warning us that we're about to do something that might be a bit risky or dangerous, or that we might not be very good at. When we feel anxious in these sorts of scenarios, we can use the feeling as a bit of a motivator. You're a smart person: you can weigh up the pros and cons for yourself. You can work out whether you're comfortable with the risk or not. You don't have to do everything that your feelings of anxiety tell you to do (or not to do). In these instances, anxiety is sort of like a little pal on your shoulder who's keeping an eye out for you, but is also a bit on the scaredy-cat side. You can usually just give it a little wave and say, 'Thanks for the warning, mate,' then carry right on with giving that new thing a go.

However, sometimes anxiety can boil over and become a full-on tyrant. It completely takes over everything. It's not a feeling of 'being a bit anxious' any more. It's Anxiety with a capital A, and it can be a real pain in the you-know-

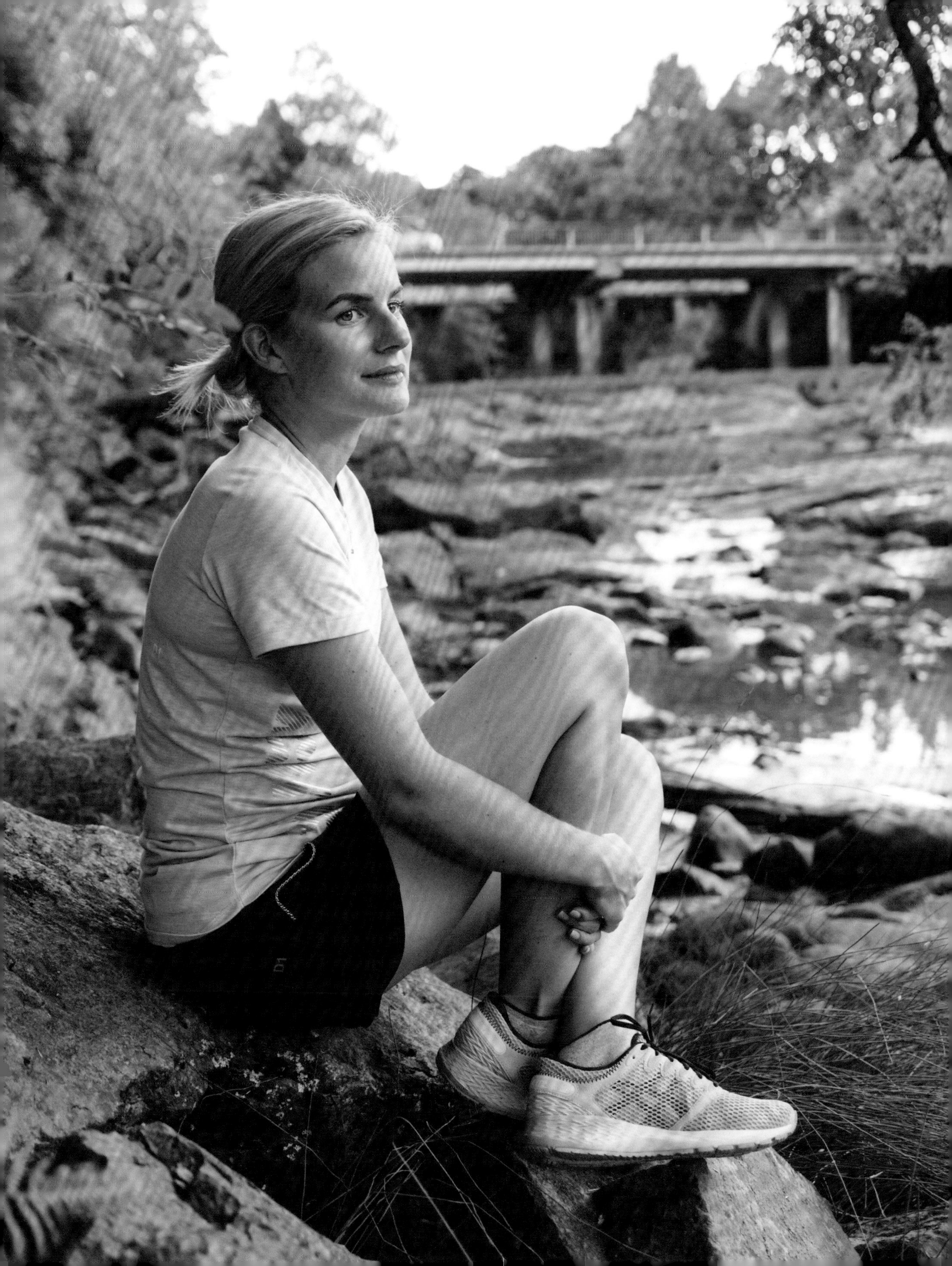

I learnt that the power of accepting myself and the current moment, warts and all, was a huge aspect of dealing with my anxiety.

what. In this case, anxiety becomes so completely overwhelming that it can make just getting through everyday life a real struggle. Anxiety gets its claws in and everything becomes too much. If you are experiencing this sort of anxiety, I'm so sorry you're going through that. I know a little bit about how you feel. A few years ago, when I was living in London, I was leading quite an unhealthy lifestyle, and my anxiety was at an all-time high. I couldn't put it down to one thing, and it was probably actually exacerbated by a whole range of things— my visa was set to expire, I had really low self-esteem, a terrible diet and felt isolated from my friends and family.

My anxiety manifested itself in many ways. I found it difficult to sleep, so was waking up at all hours. Not surprisingly, that made my work days very difficult. And, just to add to things, my childhood stutter came back with a vengeance, and that set off a vicious cycle: the stutter caused more anxiety, which caused more stuttering, which . . . Well, you get the picture. It was a terrible time. The only thing that got me through it was when I moved home and I had the support of my family. If I hadn't had that support, I would have sought professional help, because it was getting to the stage where I couldn't deal with it by myself.

If this is ringing some bells with you, or you're experiencing anxiety that feels out of control and that's having a negative impact on your life, talk to someone about it. Get professional help. You don't need to keep living like that, because there are people out there who can and will help. Don't ever be afraid to ask for help! You're not in this alone.

Once I was back home in New Zealand, I slowly started to build up my self-esteem again. I learnt that the power of accepting myself and the current moment, warts and all, was a huge aspect of dealing with my anxiety. My anxiety does still rear its ugly head from time to time, but it's usually when I've been a little slack on practising the methods in this book. I'm pretty tuned in to my body and mind these days, so I can feel when my anxiety is starting up, and I know that I need to start my practice up again.

Mindfulness can be an incredible tool when it comes to dealing with anxiety. It can help you to understand how your mind works a little better, and help you to recognise whether your anxiety is warranted or not. Most of the time, it's not.

Ever felt like you're being smothered by worry? I've been there, and it sucks. It's totally normal to think about the things that you're concerned about, but it's important to be able to realise when you're *overthinking*. Once you start overthinking, you're not doing anything that's going to help any more. In fact, it's the opposite of helpful! There's a difference between giving something thought so that you're prepared and just obsessively thinking about it, which isn't going to make an iota of difference to the outcome.

Here are some ways to recognise overthinking.

* **You're tired from thinking.** This is really common. You might feel exhausted from analysing everything in your mind, even if you haven't actually done anything physical. It's a sure-fire sign that you're allocating too much thought to something.

* **You find it hard to commit.** Being commitment-phobic is a great example of overthinking, as it's often because you're constantly worrying about the future and what might happen, and essentially talking yourself out of any commitment.

* **You're taking other people's opinions too seriously.** Overthinkers can obsessively analyse other people's words in an attempt to understand their exact meaning. Sometimes, there's no 'exact' meaning. You just need to take things at face value.

* **You can't sleep.** Ever found yourself lying in bed unable to sleep because your mind is in overdrive? Your brain should be able to

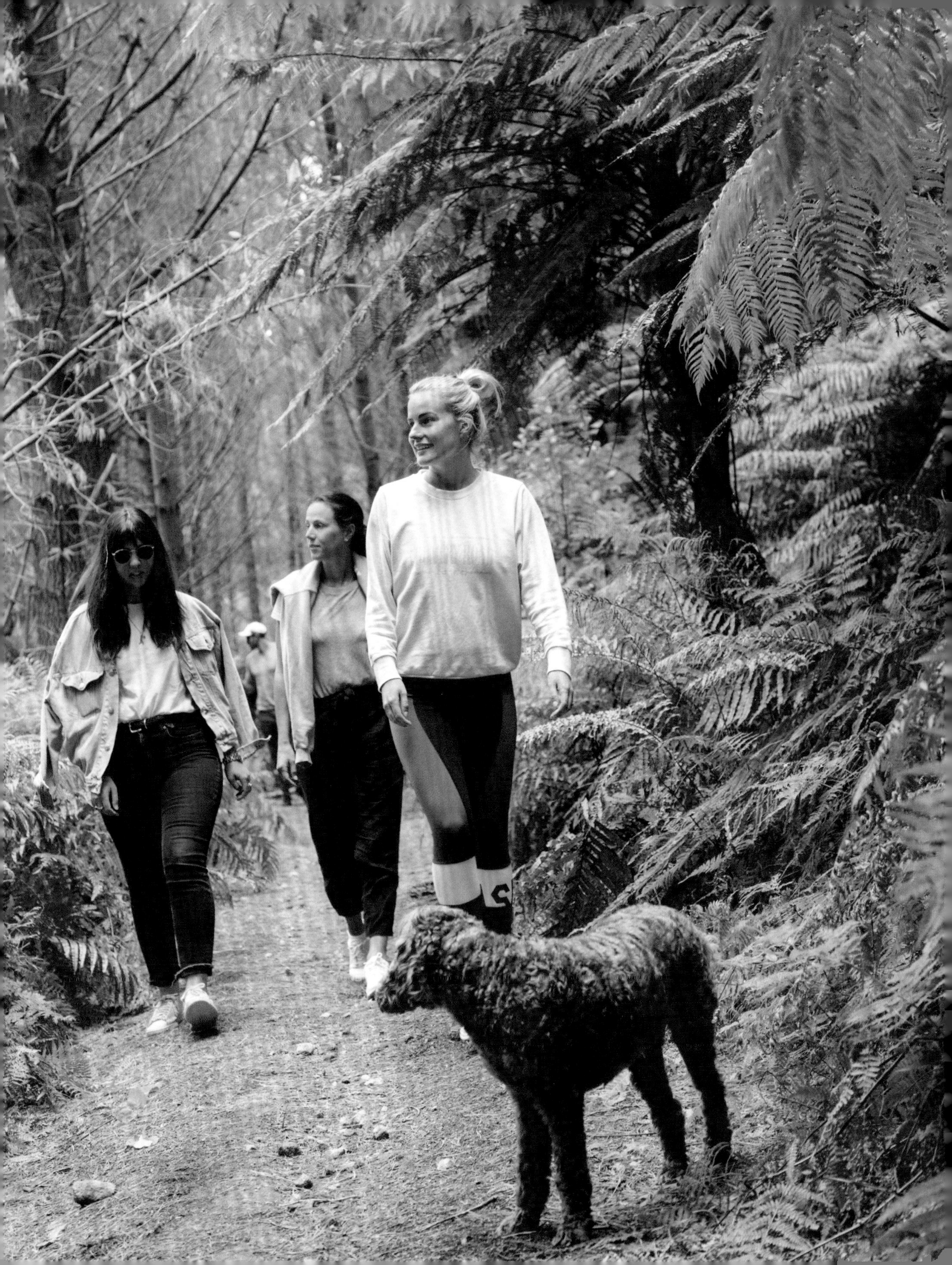

Giving too much meaning
to our thoughts can
lead us to judge not just
ourselves but others as well.
Mindfulness helps us not
to put so much weight on
our thoughts by teaching
us to realise that thoughts
are just that—thoughts.

turn off pretty easily at sleep-time. If it becomes difficult to sleep all the time—not just a one-off here and there—then, I hate to tell you, but you're possibly overthinking.

Bringing attention and awareness to all the worries and negativity we can cultivate in our own minds is important. It offers us the chance to learn to simply observe our worries and negativity, which allows us to experience unpleasant thoughts without letting those thoughts become who we are.

THE BENEFITS OF MINDFULNESS

Accepting the present moment without judgement is the key to mindfulness. We often judge ourselves based on the thoughts we have, but as soon as we learn how to simply observe these thoughts and accept them, then we can stop judging ourselves.

Giving too much meaning to our thoughts can lead us to judge not just ourselves but others as well. Mindfulness helps us not to put so much weight on our thoughts by teaching us to realise that thoughts are just that—thoughts. It teaches us to be open to whatever thoughts come into our minds and to just as easily let them go again.

In my experience, mindfulness actually sets a pretty impressive wee chain of events into action. It can go something like this:

* As you create distance between yourself and your thoughts, you'll open up more space within yourself to grow.

* In this space, you'll find the capacity to accept yourself exactly as you are, thus letting your self-esteem grow too.

* When you stop judging your thoughts, you'll also stop dwelling so much on what you perceive as your negative traits. In doing so, you'll free up more time to tap into your strengths instead—both the ones you know you have, and the ones you've yet to discover!

* As you discover and embrace your strengths, you'll notice your confidence growing. You'll open up the potential in yourself to tackle tasks and grab opportunities that you might have passed up otherwise.

* This confidence will fill you with a sense of pride that boosts your self-esteem even further.

Quite cool, huh?

What's more, mindfulness has been shown by some studies to have a positive impact on a person's sense of self, including a healthier body image, better self-esteem and resilience to negative feedback. One study even showed that practising mindful meditation boosts our immune system's ability to fight off illness.

If mindfulness was a person, it would be the best superhero known to humankind.

MINDFULNESS MEDITATION

Meditation and mindfulness kind of go hand in hand. Meditation is the main tool that all the mindfulness experts suggest. I've already talked about some of the different types of meditation, and their benefits, in the previous chapter, so flick back to that if you need a refresher.

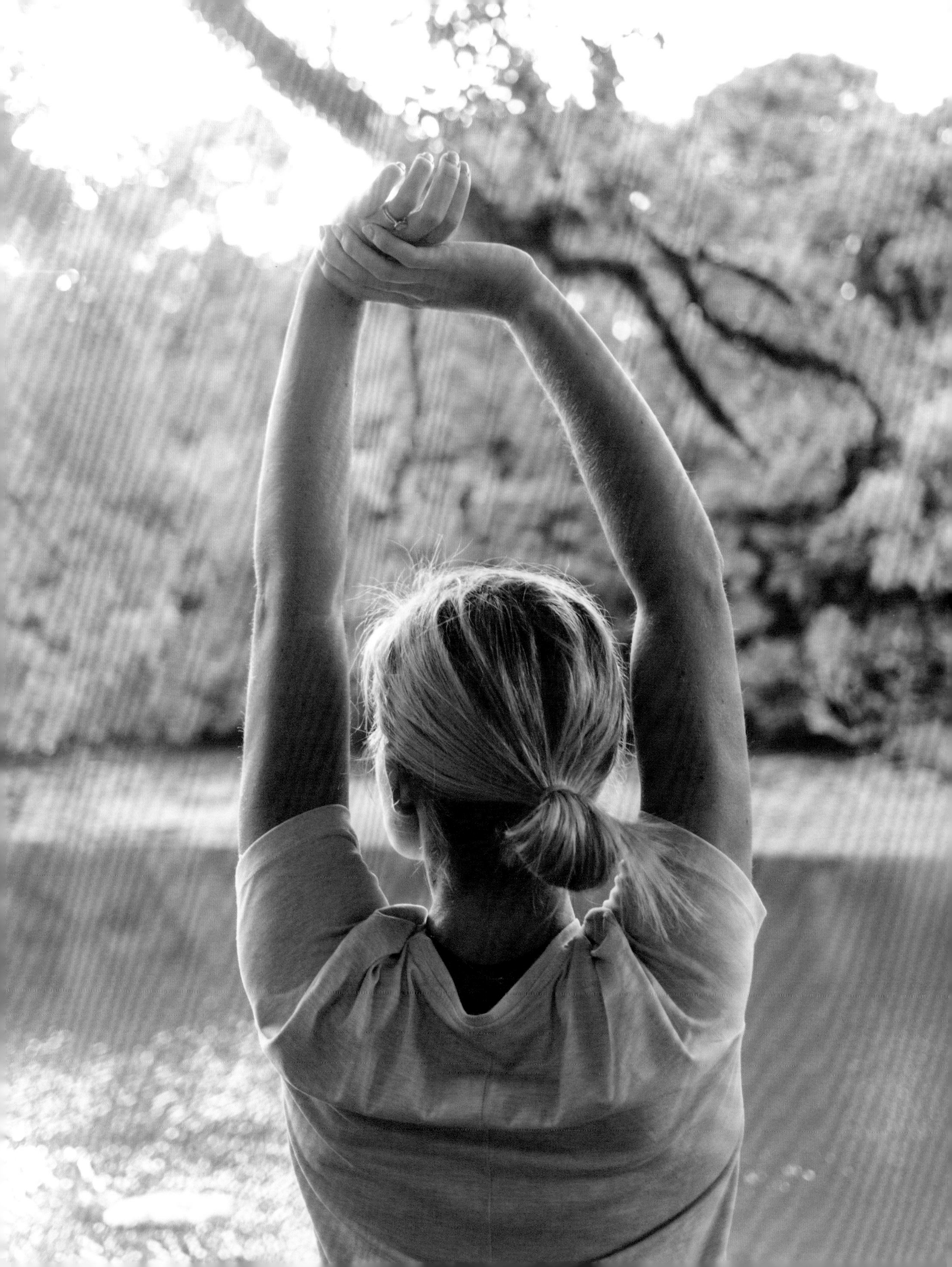

A great way to practise meditation and mindfulness together is to do 'mindful meditation' (funnily enough). This is a type of meditation designed to focus your awareness back to the current moment, rather than dwelling upon the past or the future. Insight Timer (insighttimer.com) is a great app for this one, as you can search for the type of meditation you're after.

When it comes to embarking on your mindfulness practice, take a tip from an insider: start when things are good in your life. That way, you'll be prepared when things are bad (which happens, because we're all human and that's just life).

I hope this chapter has helped to make mindfulness a little clearer to you! I know it's a complex topic, and some aspects are subjective, so just feel free to tweak things to make it your own version of what mindfulness is to you. It needs to work for you, and for it to work you have to believe in it.

When it comes to embarking on your mindfulness practice, take a tip from an insider: start when things are good in your life. That way, you'll be prepared when things are bad.

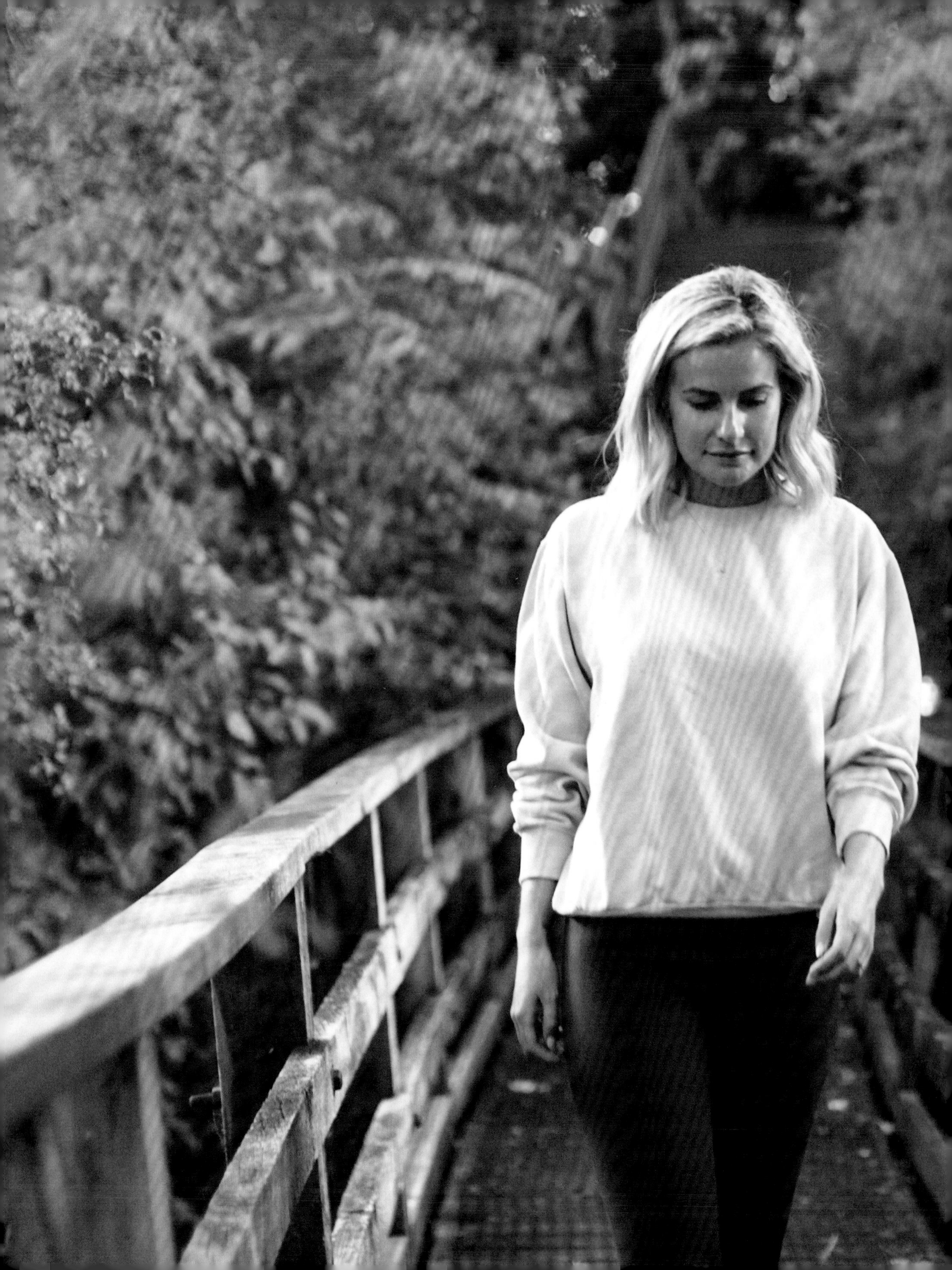

THE MINDFULNESS ACTION PLAN

✳ Start to pay attention—even to the seemingly banal everyday things like brushing your teeth, sending emails and making the bed. Get in the habit of paying attention to what you're doing and trying to stop your mind from wandering.

✳ Meditate. I won't go on about it—I've already done that in a whole other chapter! Check out page 81 for lots of information on all things meditation.

✳ Get grounded. Go outside, and get into nature. Take in the sounds, smells and feeling of everything around you. I find that, whenever I do this, I feel at my most creative. (I do need to do it more, but sometimes I just let life get in the way. That happens, though. I try not to be too hard on myself.)

✳ Check in with your five senses five times a day. This is another one I learnt from my friend Jimi, who is a huge advocate for mindfulness practices. The idea is to stop what you're doing and try to connect with your five senses—sight, smell, sound, taste and touch. Just notice how you feel, the things you can see and hear, the aromas you're smelling, how your body feels and what you can taste. Do this five times a day—or whenever you remember. It's a great way to bring your mind back to the present moment.

✳ Breathe. Take a few deep breaths down into your tummy (not your chest). This is called diaphragmatic breathing, and it has a profound effect. It's even been suggested that it can calm down your nervous system.

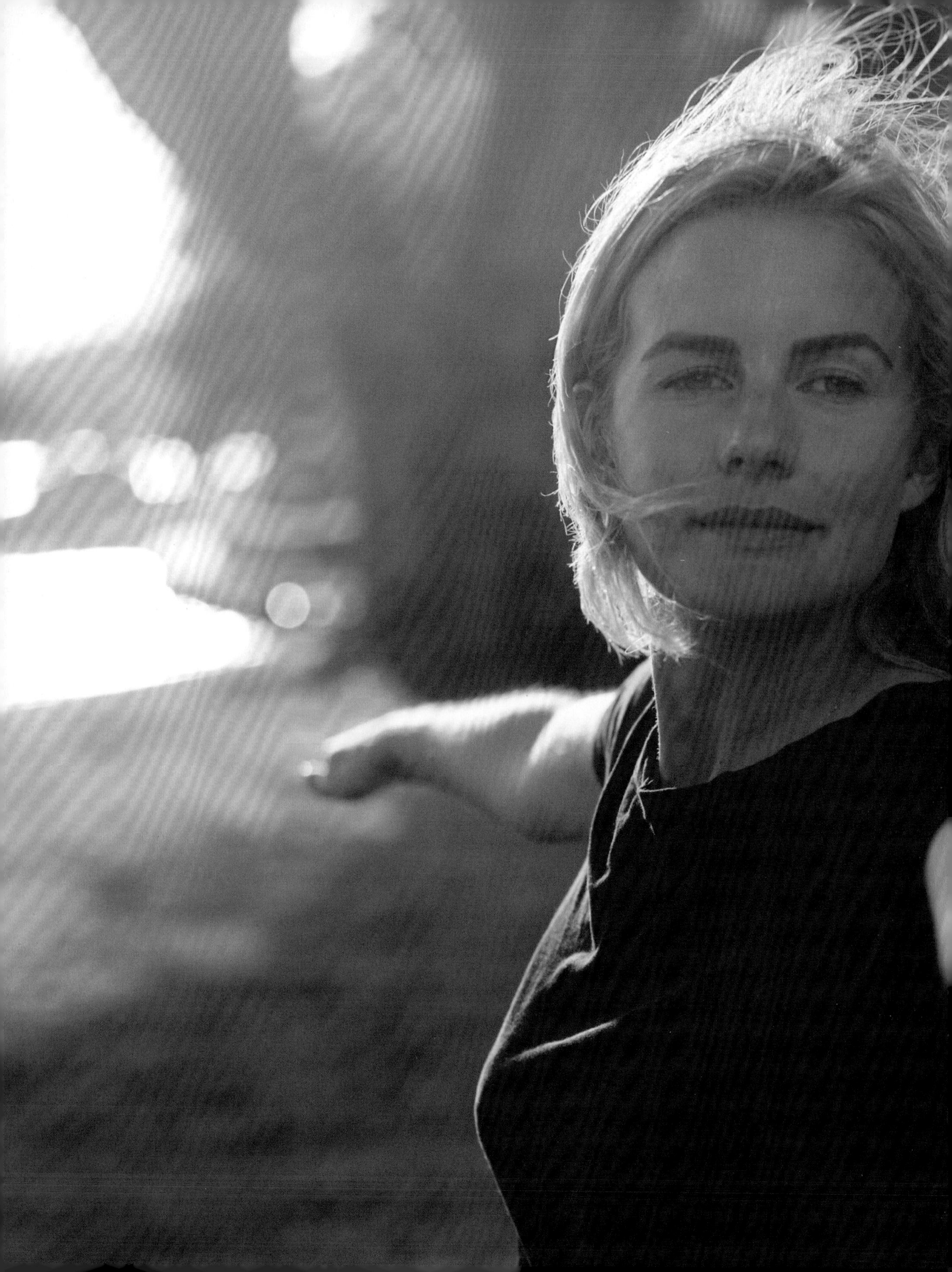

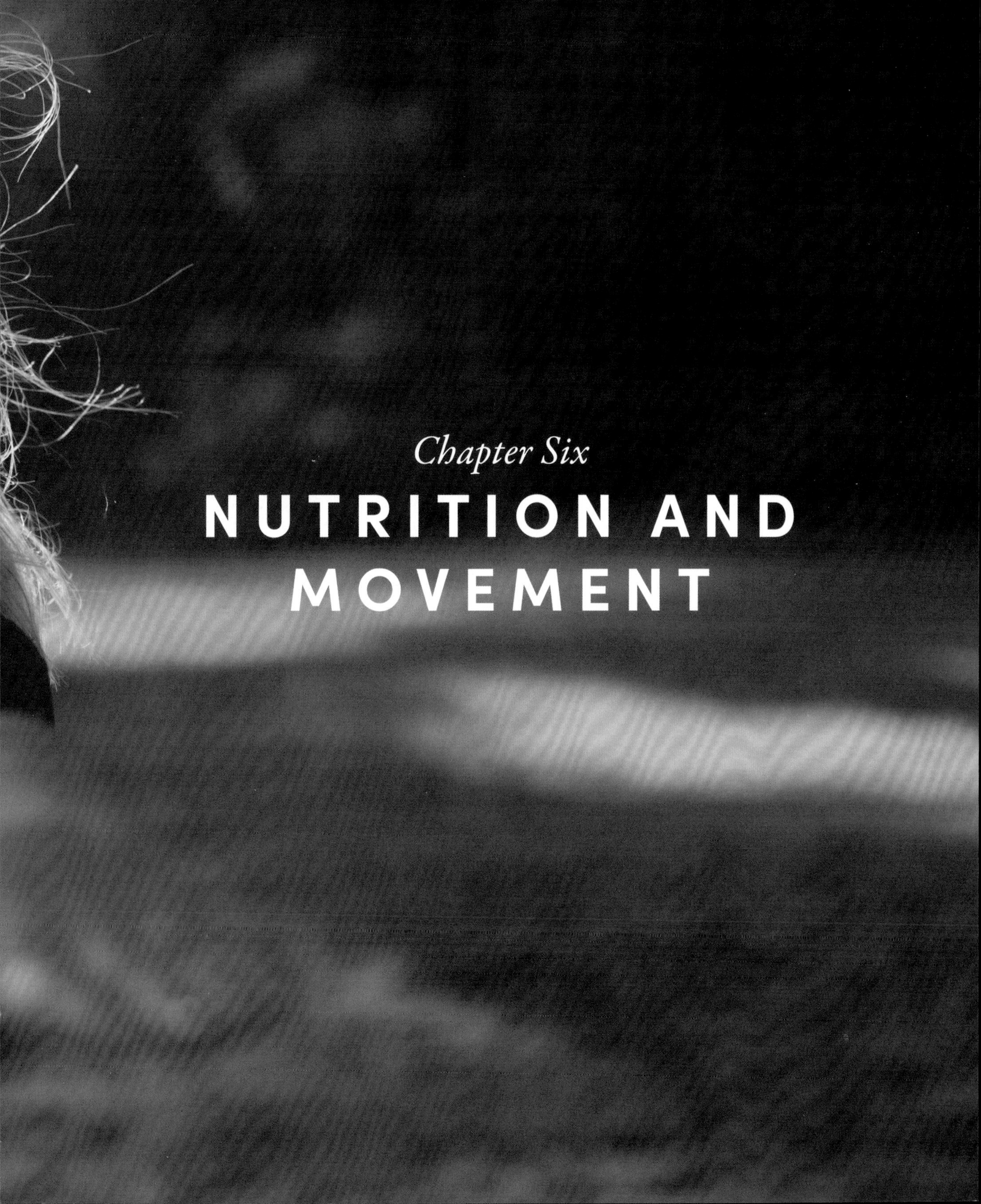

Chapter Six

NUTRITION AND MOVEMENT

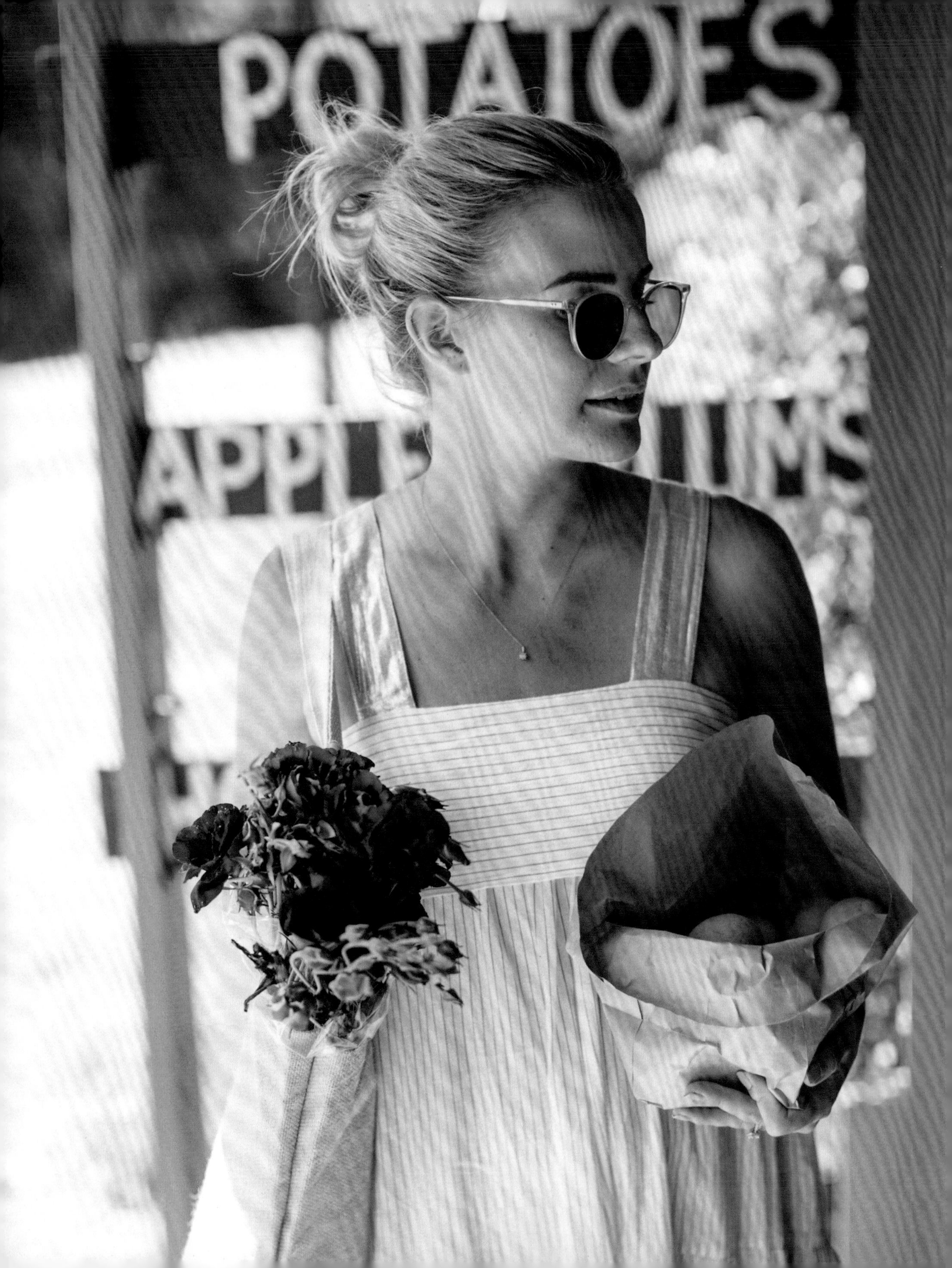
POTATOES

So far, we've covered a whole bunch of neat tricks for taking care of your mind and your soul, but there's another (much more obvious) way you can take care of yourself, and that's through nutrition. There's that old saying that you are what you eat, and when it comes to self-esteem this is actually pretty spot on. The food we eat has a massive impact on how we feel, so what you are or aren't eating might be affecting your self-esteem and your general mood more than you know. And it's not just about *what* you eat, either; it also has a heap to do with how you *feel* about what you're eating and about yourself.

Let's get one thing straight, though: I'm not talking about going on some super-restrictive diet, or about changing your body, because I already know it's perfect the way it is. Remember when I said way back at the start of this book that I wouldn't dream of asking you to change who you are? Well, I meant it. You're already perfect the way you are. We are all born different from one another, and building good self-esteem starts from a place of accepting— actually, loving!—that difference.

What I am talking about is cultivating a healthy relationship with your body and with the stuff you put into it. That doesn't mean you *never* eat certain foods, or that you go around labelling food as either 'good' or 'bad'. It means being in touch with what's going to make you feel great about yourself, and trying to avoid the stuff that will have the opposite effect. It means enjoying your food, and enjoying your amazing body and all the incredible things it does for you.

I know that having a healthy relationship with food and your body is, sadly, the exception rather than the norm these days. If you're anything like me, you'll have had your own moments when you weren't a fan of your body, and you may have wanted to force it to change by—to be blunt—not being very kind to it. I've done lots of restrictive diets in the past, cutting out everything from carbohydrates to sugar to heavily cutting calories. Doing some of these things did make me lose weight, but at what cost? I can tell you I certainly wasn't happy. Oh no, far from it. The more I tried to change myself, the unhappier I became. Any time I indulged in something delicious that wasn't part of my 'diet plan', I would be plagued with guilt and feel really anxious. That's no way to live. Food is one of the most incredible pleasures in life! It's social, and fun. It's creative. It's just the bloody best! Your relationship with food should be one of love, not guilt.

If you are currently engaged in a war with your own body, I'm so sorry to hear that, and I want to hug you, because I know how it feels. So, please just imagine I'm hugging you through this book. And let me tell you something you might not have realised: you are so beautiful exactly the way that you are. Please know that you don't have to change yourself or how you look. Please know that how good a person you are inside has zilch to do with what you look like on the outside. Please know that you have an absolutely incredible body, and it—just like you—deserves to be loved. There's so much pressure on us from every angle to look a certain way, and to eat or not eat certain things, that it's understandable that lots of us just end up feeling like total failures when we're not at all.

When it comes to feeling good about yourself, I believe that forming a healthy relationship with both your body and what you're putting into it is one

Food is one of the most incredible pleasures in life! It's social, and fun. It's creative. It's just the bloody best! Your relationship with food should be one of love, not guilt.

of those self-esteem foundation stones I talked about earlier. It's not necessarily something that comes naturally, but it's definitely something you can learn to be aware of and spend time nurturing. Simply put, in order to nourish your self-esteem, I believe it's also important to nourish your body.

So, in this chapter, I'm going to spend some time talking about my own nutrition philosophy, and how that contributes to me feeling all-round tip-top in both mind and body.

MY NUTRITION PHILOSOPHY

For the past couple of years, I've been using an 'unprocessed/wholefood' philosophy when it comes to food, and I have definitely experienced positive results—which I'll talk about in more detail below. When I use the term 'wholefood', what I essentially mean is that the food is in its most natural state, with the least amount of refining or processing and no additives. Basically, if food comes from the ground or a paddock and has been 'tampered with' as little as possible, then it's good to eat in my eyes.

A great tip of Art's is to get 90 per cent of your groceries from the outside aisles of the supermarket—you know, the ones where all the fresh veggies and fruit, meat, seafood, eggs and dairy are found. Delve into those middle aisles for no more than 10 per cent of your food. The middle aisles are where you tend to find packaged and processed foods, and these foods might potentially cause your body the most harm—whether it's cos they're loaded with highly refined carbohydrates and sugars or chock-full of ingredients like preservatives, colours and flavours. Or just numbers.

I also like to avoid anything with ingredients that are so sciency sounding that I feel like I need to go to university and get a science degree just to understand them. If you're confused about labels on packaged food, here's a great rule of thumb: if you don't know what an ingredient on the label

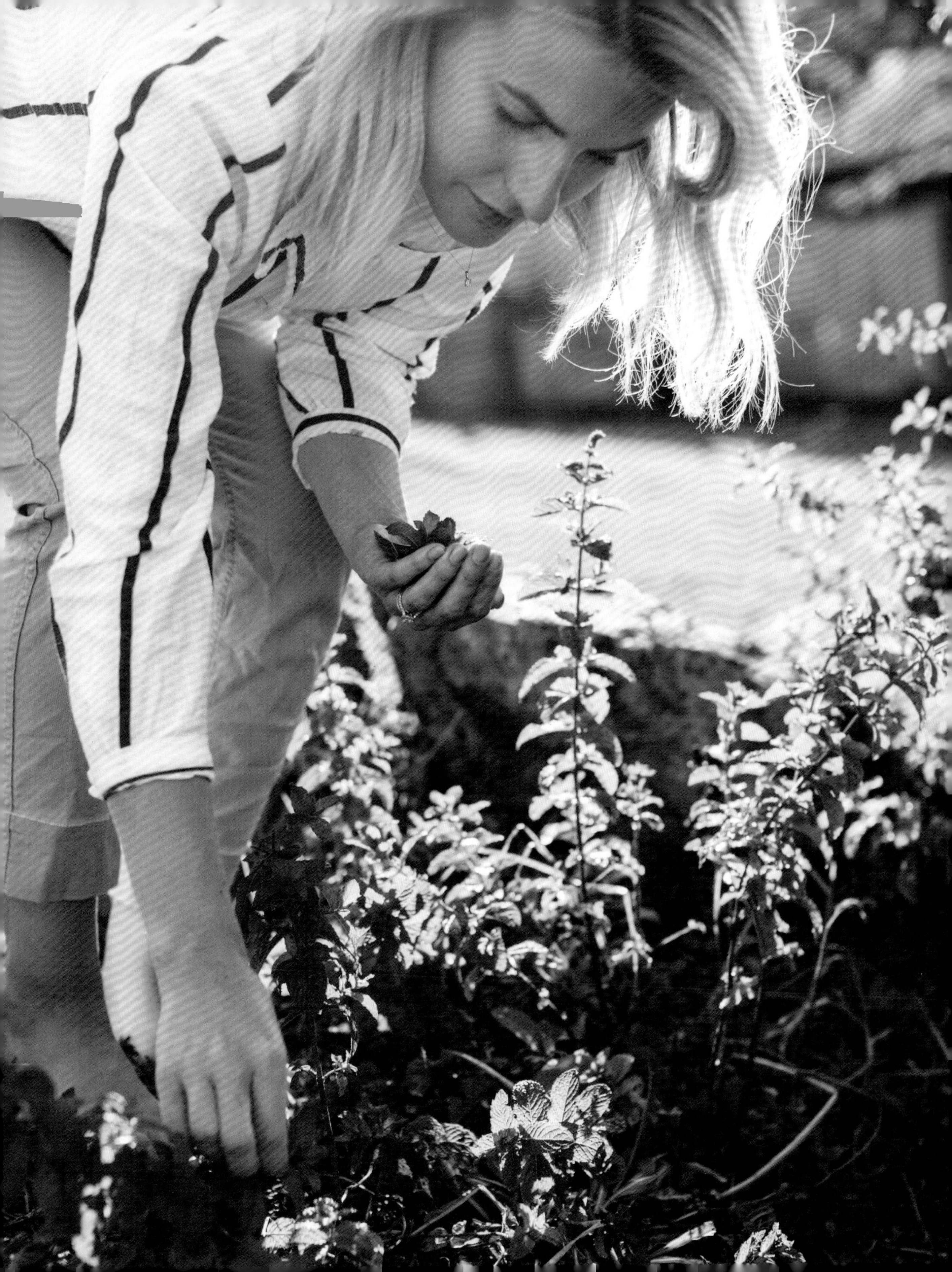

When I eat better, I feel better, and when I feel better, I look better. And when I say 'look better', I'm not talking about weight; I mean my skin improves and anxiety decreases, and that in turn can increase my confidence and my self-esteem.

is, don't buy it. You could spend hours googling ingredients while you're standing in the supermarket, or you could save yourself time and just buy food that has recognisable ingredients in there—or, in other words, buy food that is actually food.

EAT GOOD, FEEL GOOD

When I started to eat healthy, unprocessed foods, it wasn't long before I started to feel better in so many ways. Among other things, I have more energy and generally a more positive outlook on life. I even sleep better.

The proof is in the pudding. (Bad pun. Sorry.) For me, it basically goes something like this: when I eat better, I feel better, and when I feel better, I look better. And when I say 'look better', I'm not talking about weight; I mean my skin improves and anxiety decreases, and that in turn can increase my confidence and my self-esteem. I've always liked the analogy that your body is like a car. If you look after your car, get it serviced on time, drive it regularly, keep it clean, use premium fuel, it's going to run better and last longer.

That saying that you are what you eat, which I mentioned earlier, has actually been found to have some truth to it. You know your cells? Those tiny little building blocks that make up everything in your entire body (at least, that's my non-scientific definition)? Well, keeping them healthy is essential! The average person has approximately 30 trillion cells in their body (give or take a few mill, perhaps). They are constantly dying due to damage or old age, which is completely normal, and being replaced by brand-new cells. The nutrition you get from the food you eat goes towards the new cells, so there's a pretty good incentive to eat lots of healthy wholefoods. Think of the cells, people!

Cells also have these tiny internal structures called organelles that do most of the day-to-day cell stuff. One of the most important organelles is the mitochondrion. (Sorry, other organelles, you're important too, I promise.) Mitochondria basically act like the digestive system in your cells—they're what keep your cells full of energy from the food you've been eating. Your mitochondria are really important to your overall health and well-being, so you wanna be fuelling them with the good stuff.

TOO SUGARY SWEET

In 2015, a post titled 'Nutritional Psychiatry: Your brain on food' published on the Harvard Medical School blog, noted that multiple studies have found a correlation between diets high in refined sugars and impaired brain function, and even 'a worsening of symptoms of mood disorders, such as depression'. Scary, right?

So, what is refined sugar? It comes from sugar cane or sugar beets, which are processed to extract the sugar. Refined sugar scores incredibly high on the glycemic index (GI), which means that it causes your blood-sugar levels to spike rapidly—something that, if frequently occurring, can cause your body to store fat and, potentially, develop diabetes. Nowadays, we also have a whole list of refined sugars that food manufacturers hide behind other names: things like high-fructose corn syrup, sucrose, barley malt, dextrose, maltose, rice syrup . . . The list goes on. Literally. This is why it pays to read the ingredients labels on the food you're buying.

While I don't eliminate anything from my diet completely, I do try to limit refined sugar as much as possible, because it can cause negative effects if you have too much. However, a healthy and balanced diet does include treats. As long as you're mostly eating lots of fresh wholefoods, then a bit of junk food every once in a while won't hurt. Our bodies are pretty tough, and I believe that it's what we do most of the time—not some of the time—that has a long-term effect on us. So I'm not saying to NEVER eat sugar. Just be conscious

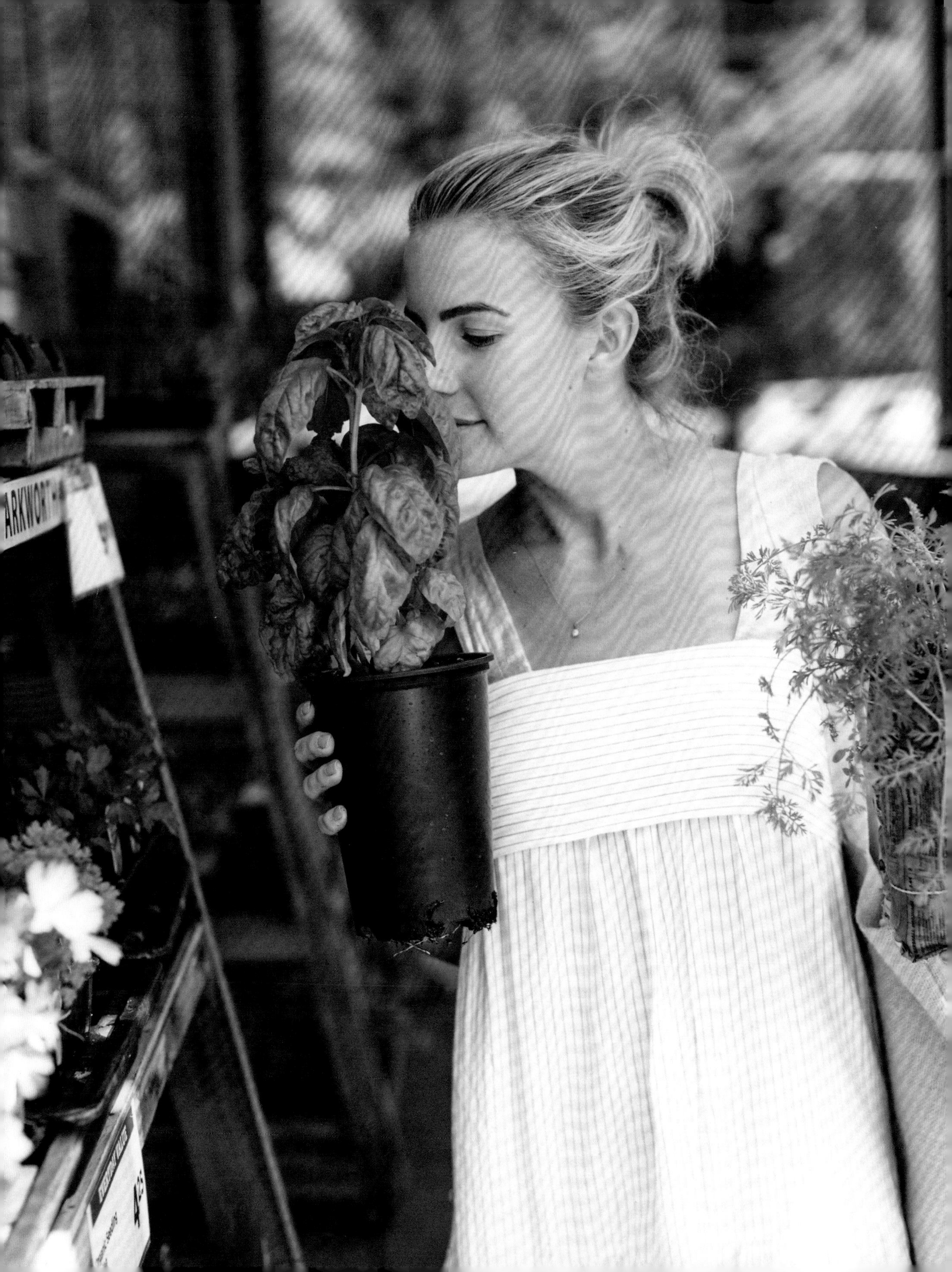
ARKWORT

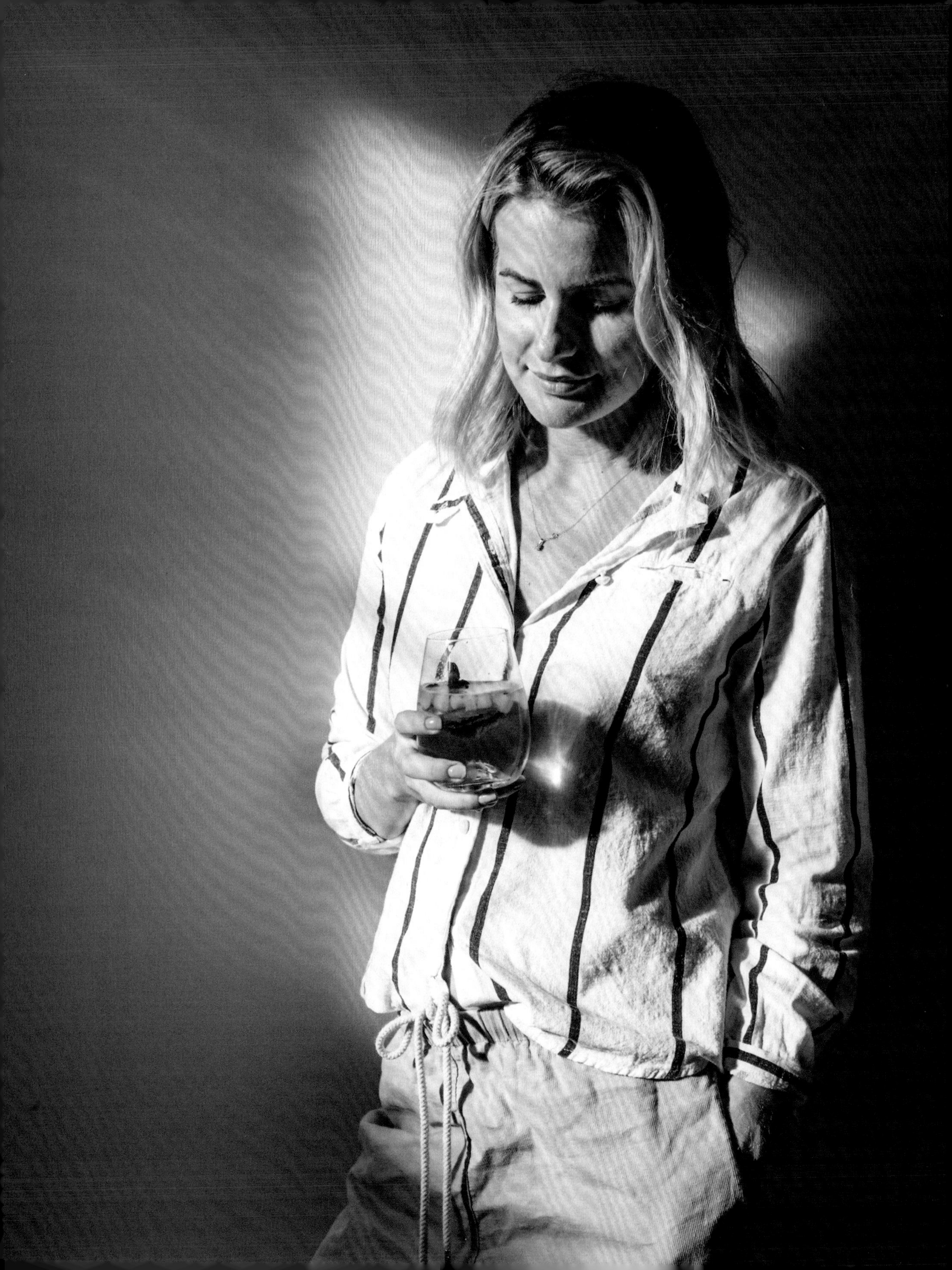

of how much sugar you are really eating, because it's often hidden—and manufacturers will go to great lengths to trick you into thinking it's not there. Be aware and informed about what's really in your food.

As a side note, you should also watch out for trans fats, which is short for 'trans fatty acids'. This is the type of fat that also gets called 'bad fat' (as opposed to the good kind, like olive oil and avocados, which healthy diets tend to include). Trans fats are actually so bad that they're banned in the US! In 2013, the Food and Drug Administration (FDA) ruled that artificial trans fats were unsafe to eat, and gave food producers until June 2018 to eliminate them from the food supply.

But, back to the sweet stuff. 'What about artificial sugar?' I hear you ask. Well, unfortunately, some research has suggested that artificial sugar can actually be just as bad as refined sugar. One US study assessed data from the Multi-Ethnic Study of Atherosclerosis (MESA) and found that consumption of diet soda at least daily was associated with significantly greater risks of 'select incident metabolic syndrome components' and type 2 diabetes. Unfortunately, that means that, when things on the sweetener front seem too good to be true, they probably are. You're better to just avoid fizzy drinks altogether, in my opinion (or, at least, don't have them every day). Have some water instead.

So far we've talked about refined sugar and artificial sugar, but there are other forms of sugar out there, too—sugars that come in fresh fruit, or in things like maple syrup or honey. The great thing about eating a piece of fruit is that you're getting the full nutritional picture, including all of the fibre, vitamins, minerals and other good stuff as well as the sugars. Your body can digest a piece of fruit much more efficiently than the likes of a glass of coke or a chocolate bar. The sugars in the fruit, in the form of fructose, hit your liver slowly, so it's much easier for your body to break it all down. What's more, the fibre in the fruit also helps to slow down the absorption of carbohydrates, meaning your blood sugar doesn't rise as rapidly as it would from just sugar or fructose alone.

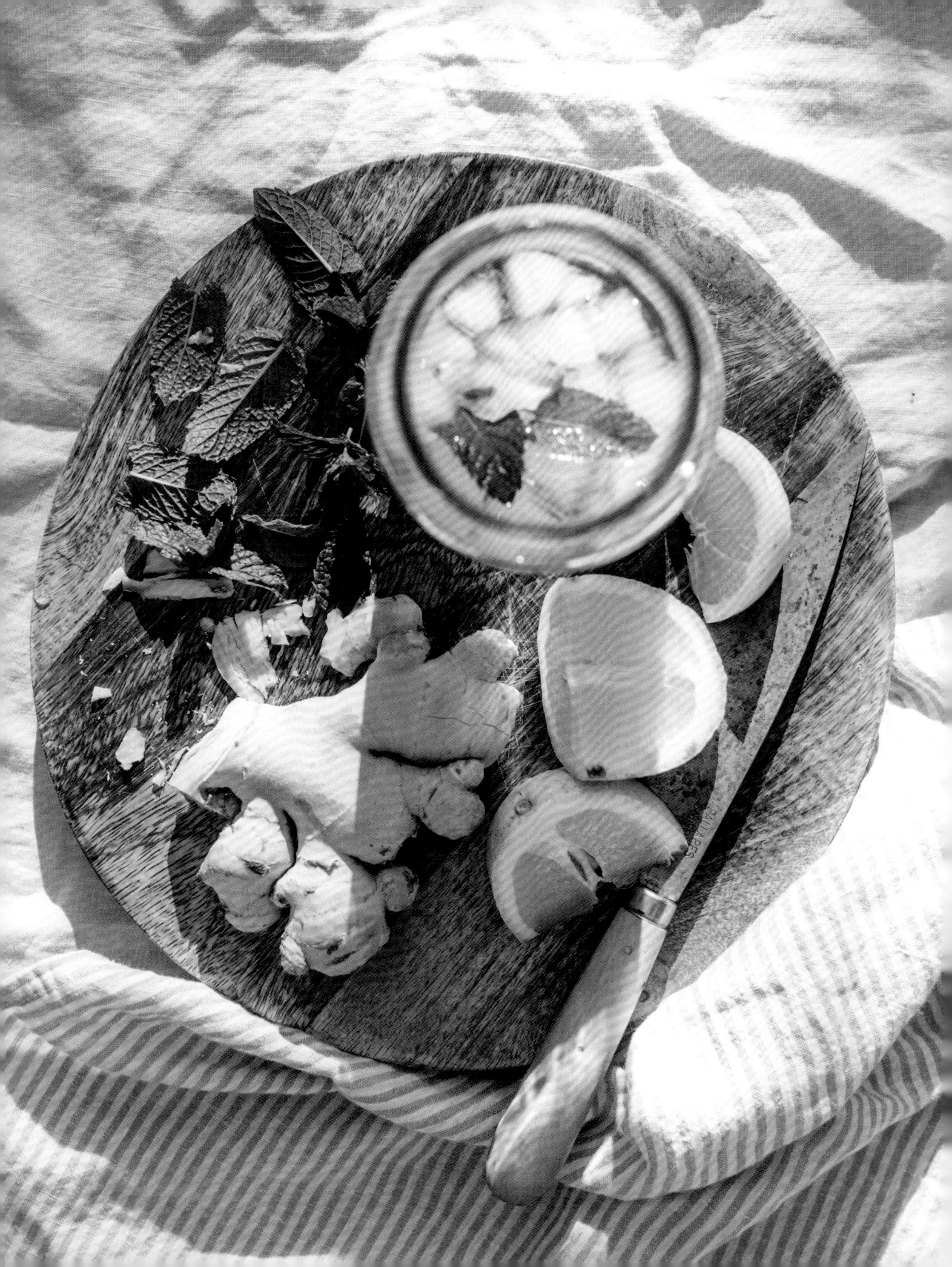

But (and there's always a but!) a fruit juice is *not* the same thing as a piece of fruit. When you juice fruit, you lose the fibre content. Plus, you tend to need a LOT of fruit just to make one glass of juice. That means you're getting more sugar in a glass of juice than you would from eating just one piece of fruit. If you've got a hankering for something sweet, you're better just to stick with a good old apple.

Keep an eye on those low-fat options, too. A lot of the time, manufacturers cut the fat content in a product by topping it up with sugar so it still tastes good. Make sure you check that ingredients label.

Another thing to be wary of if you're trying to be more aware of your sugar consumption is 'natural treats'. You know the ones I mean—things like raw cheesecake or bliss balls. These treats are a great option if you're after something natural or are sensitive to gluten or dairy, but they certainly aren't sugar free. A lot of natural treats like this use dates, honey or maple syrup, and all of these things are of course very high in sugar. You can make the argument that at least you're not having something processed, but just don't be under any illusion that you can eat a heap of these treats. They're still treats, after all. And, at the end of the day, sugar is still sugar!

NOT ALL CALORIES ARE CREATED EQUAL

There's sometimes an idea out there that 'a calorie is a calorie' and where it comes from doesn't matter, but some health experts have suggested that thinking doesn't necessarily hold true.

Dr Mark Hyman, the director at Cleveland Clinic's Center for Functional Medicine, is kind of a guru for all things health in my eyes. In a piece titled 'Why Calories Don't Matter' published on his website (drhyman.com), he dissects the common idea that all calories are created equal, and points out how this is not quite accurate. He uses the comparison of 750 calories of broccoli with 750 calories of fizzy drink. While it's true that, when tested in a laboratory, the two do produce the same amount of energy, he discusses how that kind of goes out the window as soon as you pay attention to what happens *inside* your body. According to Hyman, the fizzy drink causes your blood sugar to instantly spike and your insulin levels to go haywire, which means your brain doesn't get the 'I'm full' signal and you just end up wanting more sugar. The broccoli, on the other hand, contains so much fibre that very few of the calories actually get absorbed, and those that do are absorbed very slowly. There's no blood sugar or insulin spike, and your brain gets the 'I'm full' signal—not least from your full tummy.

So there you have it, folks—not all calories are created equal, after all. As Hyman explains, 'some calories are addictive, others healing, some fattening, some metabolism-boosting. That's because food doesn't just contain calories, it contains information.'

If all you care about is losing weight, then counting calories can be a means to an end. However, as I've already mentioned, I don't think your weight is the be all and end all when it comes to your health. It has to be a full-body approach, in my opinion. If you want to be healthy, I think it's more important to focus on the type of food you are putting into your body than on counting calories. Food is about so many things—good company, tastiness, enjoyment, feeling great—but I personally don't think it's about numbers.

MOVE YOUR BOOTY!

Exercise and nutrition go hand in hand. Like salt and pepper, Mario and Luigi, fish and chips, Ben and Jerry—all good by themselves, but bloody unstoppable when together.

Your diet and exercise regime is really important to your overall well-being. I find that, as soon as I've finished a spot of exercise, I feel instantly better—

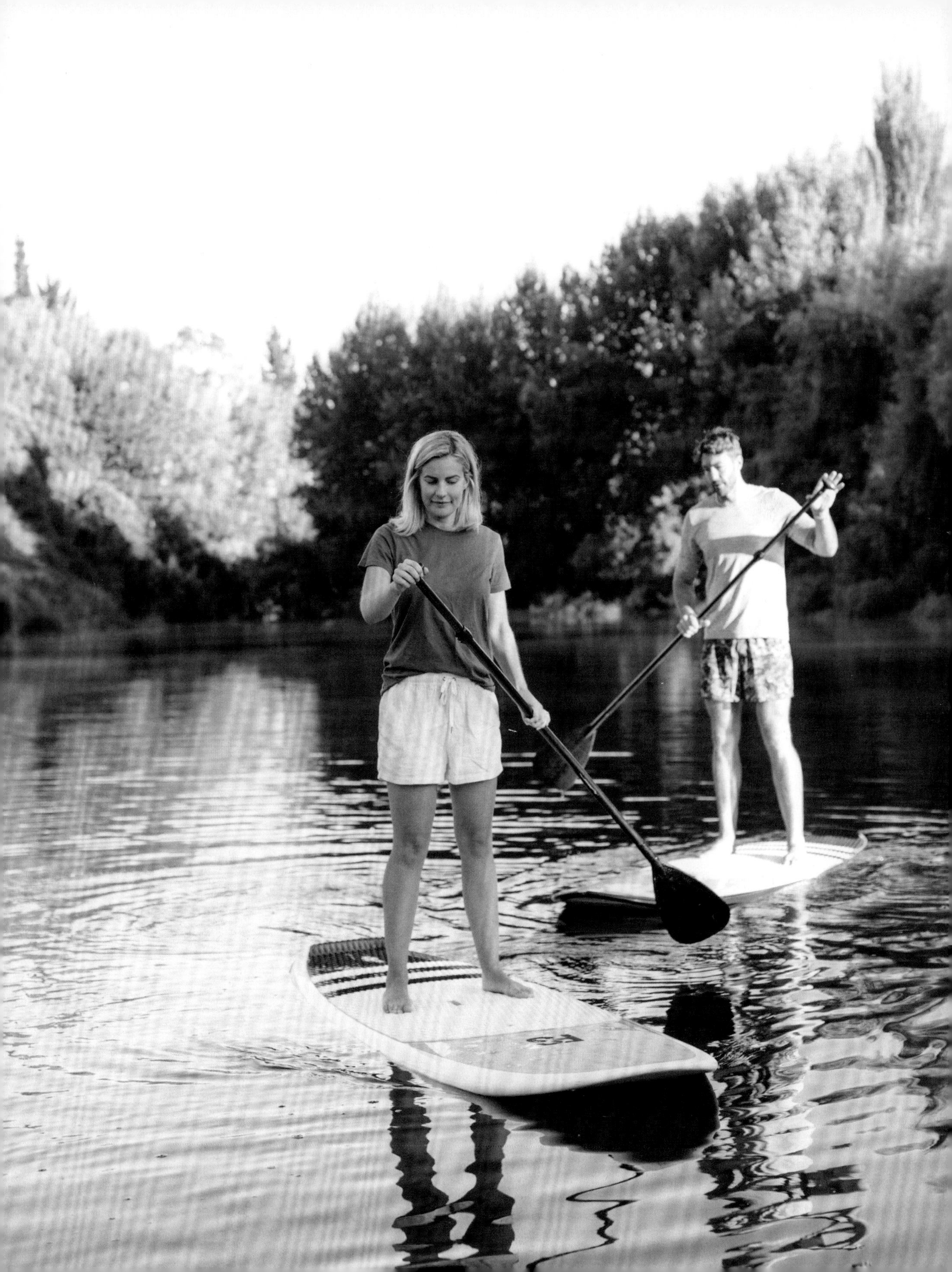

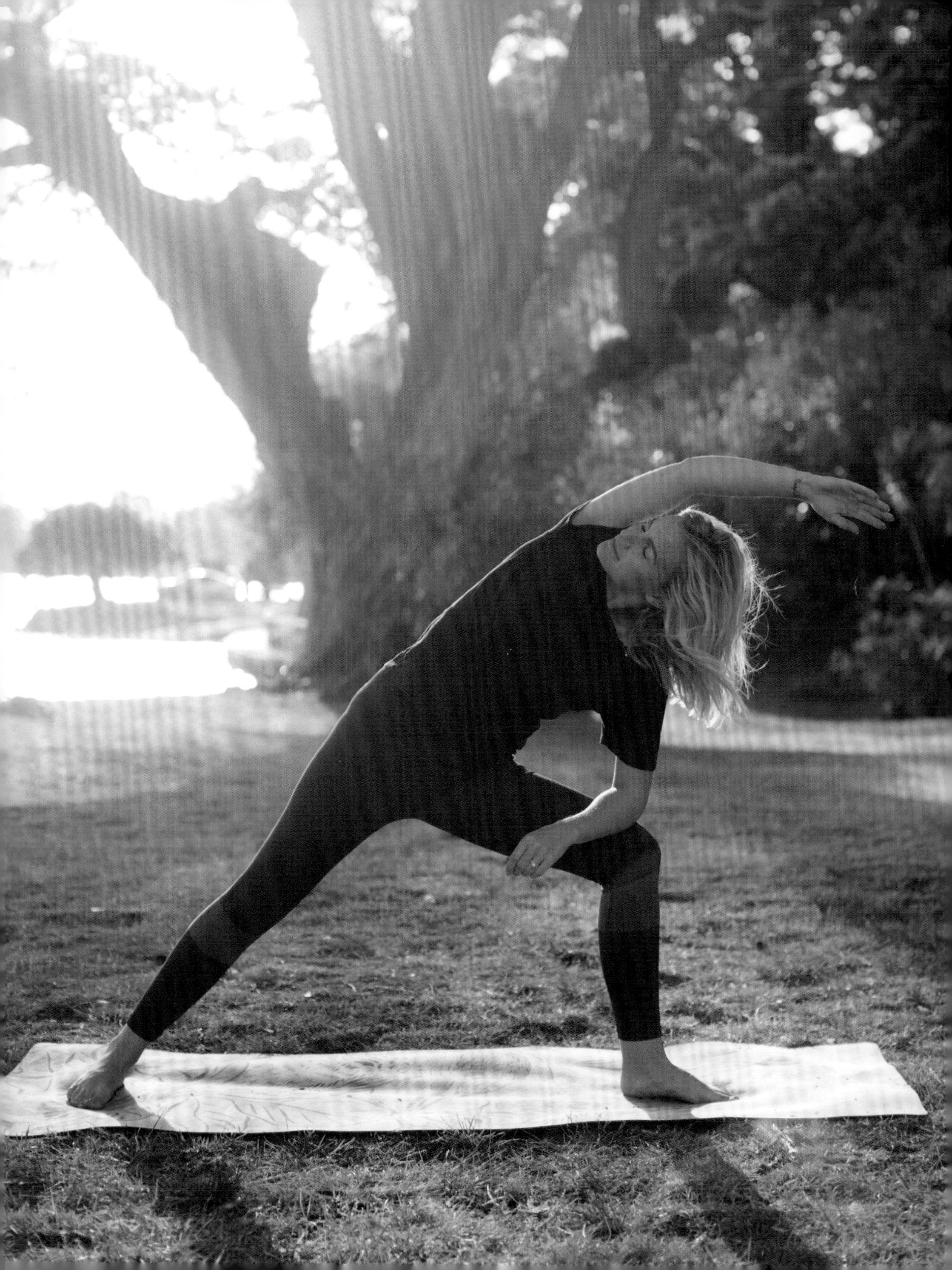

and that's even if I already felt good beforehand. Those endorphins everyone talks about are seriously legit. (Endorphins, in case you don't know, are a type of hormone in your body that basically make you feel less pain and stress, and make you feel more upbeat—in other words, a great one to boost.)

When you exercise regularly, you feel better, which in turn makes you look better. (I'm talking about the glow from the inside here, not anything superficial.) And you know what? Feeling and looking better makes you more confident, and that boosts your self-esteem. It's all pretty obvious when you put it like that, right?

I feel unstoppable when I've got a good exercise routine going, and that feeling tends to flow into all other areas of my life so that I feel like I'm on top of everything.

When it comes to exercise, do what works for you and your body. It might just be popping out to go for a stroll round the block or you might be a gym-class junkie. You might prefer doing something that doesn't even feel like exercise, like a dance class. It doesn't have to be hard out—unless you want it to be! It's really just about finding a way to move your body, to get your lungs full of air, your muscles moving and your head clear.

BE KIND TO YOUR BODY

Nutrition is so important, as it is literally the fuel that keeps you going. I know you've all heard the cliché, 'It's not a diet. It's a lifestyle.' But that quote really is spot on. A diet is often framed as a way to punish our bodies (and ourselves) for being 'naughty' and putting on weight, but a much healthier way to look at it is that 'diet' really just means 'what you eat'. A diet doesn't have to be a quick weight-loss fix.

So, instead of punishing your body, start to love it by making healthier choices that nourish it. Because, after all, your body does a hell of a lot for you—it's your one true home, you only get one, and it does try its best (even if it doesn't always feel like it). It deserves to be treated kindly, just like you do, with things that make it feel good and work efficiently. Don't fill it with junk.

At the same time, remember that life is all about balance. It can be easy to become so obsessed with the idea of filling your body with 'good' fuel, that you can end up berating yourself if you have something that's not on the 'good' list. I'd actually suggest you let go of the 'good' and 'bad' labels altogether when it comes to food, because they're just not helpful. Remember that moderation is the key to everything. I've said it once and I'll say it again: it's what you do most of the time that matters, not what you do every now and then. When I say 'look after your body', I mean you should also indulge in treats once in a while if you have a hankering. Your mental health is just as important as your physical health, so cut yourself some slack. We're all human! The most powerful thing you can do is to be kind to yourself.

Your mental health is just as important as your physical health, so cut yourself some slack. We're all human! The most powerful thing you can do is to be kind to yourself.

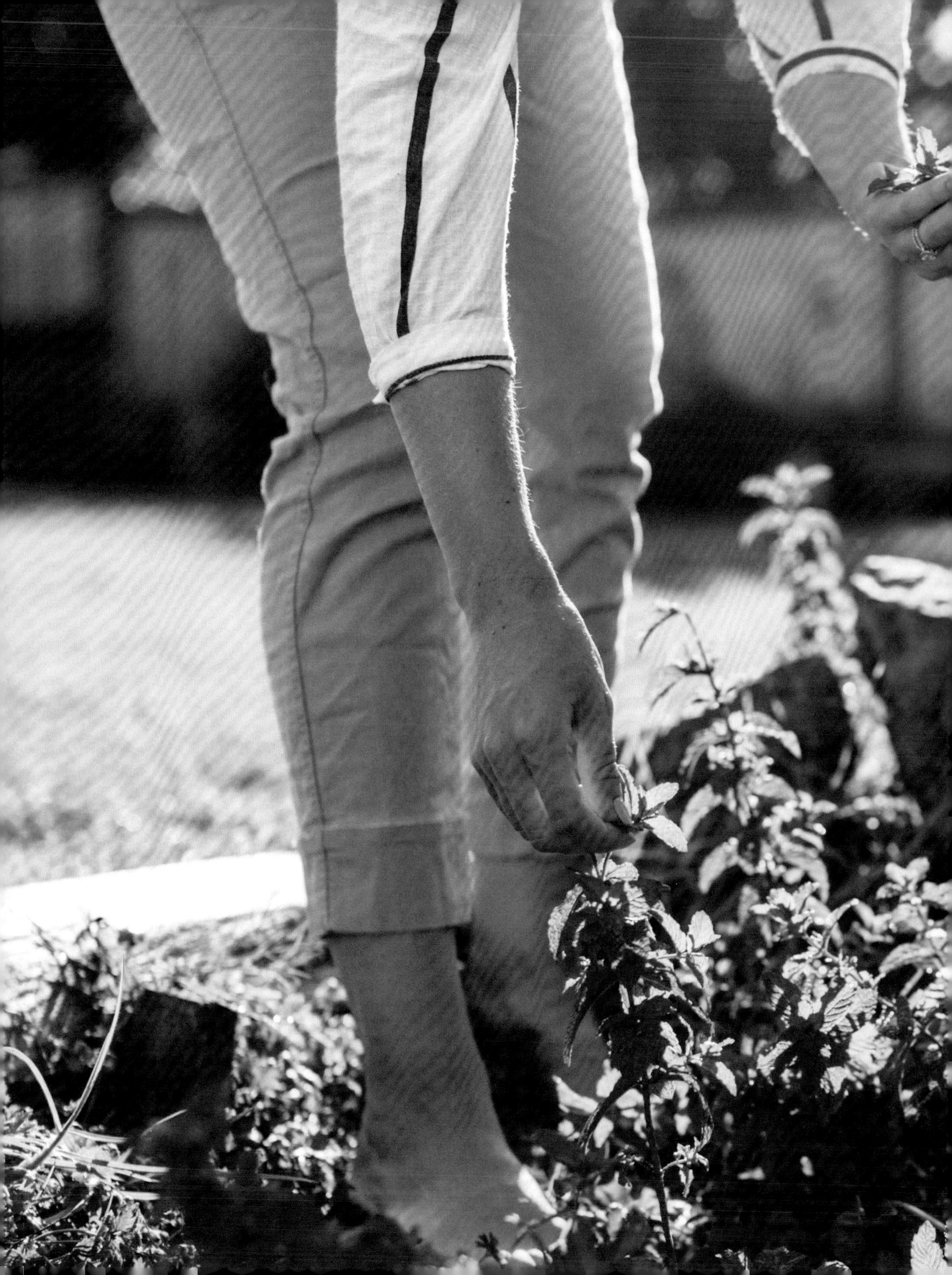

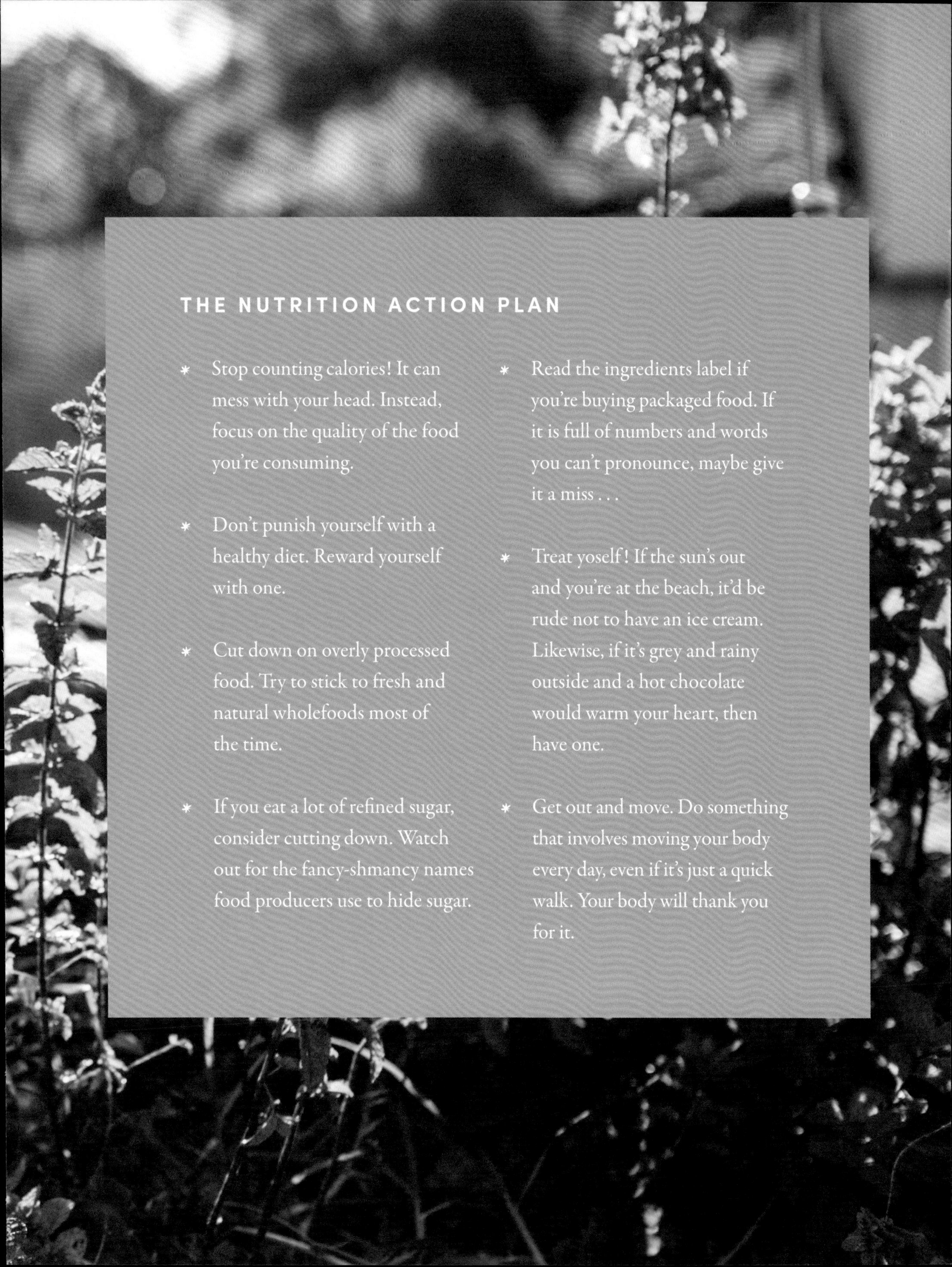

THE NUTRITION ACTION PLAN

* Stop counting calories! It can mess with your head. Instead, focus on the quality of the food you're consuming.
* Don't punish yourself with a healthy diet. Reward yourself with one.
* Cut down on overly processed food. Try to stick to fresh and natural wholefoods most of the time.
* If you eat a lot of refined sugar, consider cutting down. Watch out for the fancy-shmancy names food producers use to hide sugar.
* Read the ingredients label if you're buying packaged food. If it is full of numbers and words you can't pronounce, maybe give it a miss . . .
* Treat yoself! If the sun's out and you're at the beach, it'd be rude not to have an ice cream. Likewise, if it's grey and rainy outside and a hot chocolate would warm your heart, then have one.
* Get out and move. Do something that involves moving your body every day, even if it's just a quick walk. Your body will thank you for it.

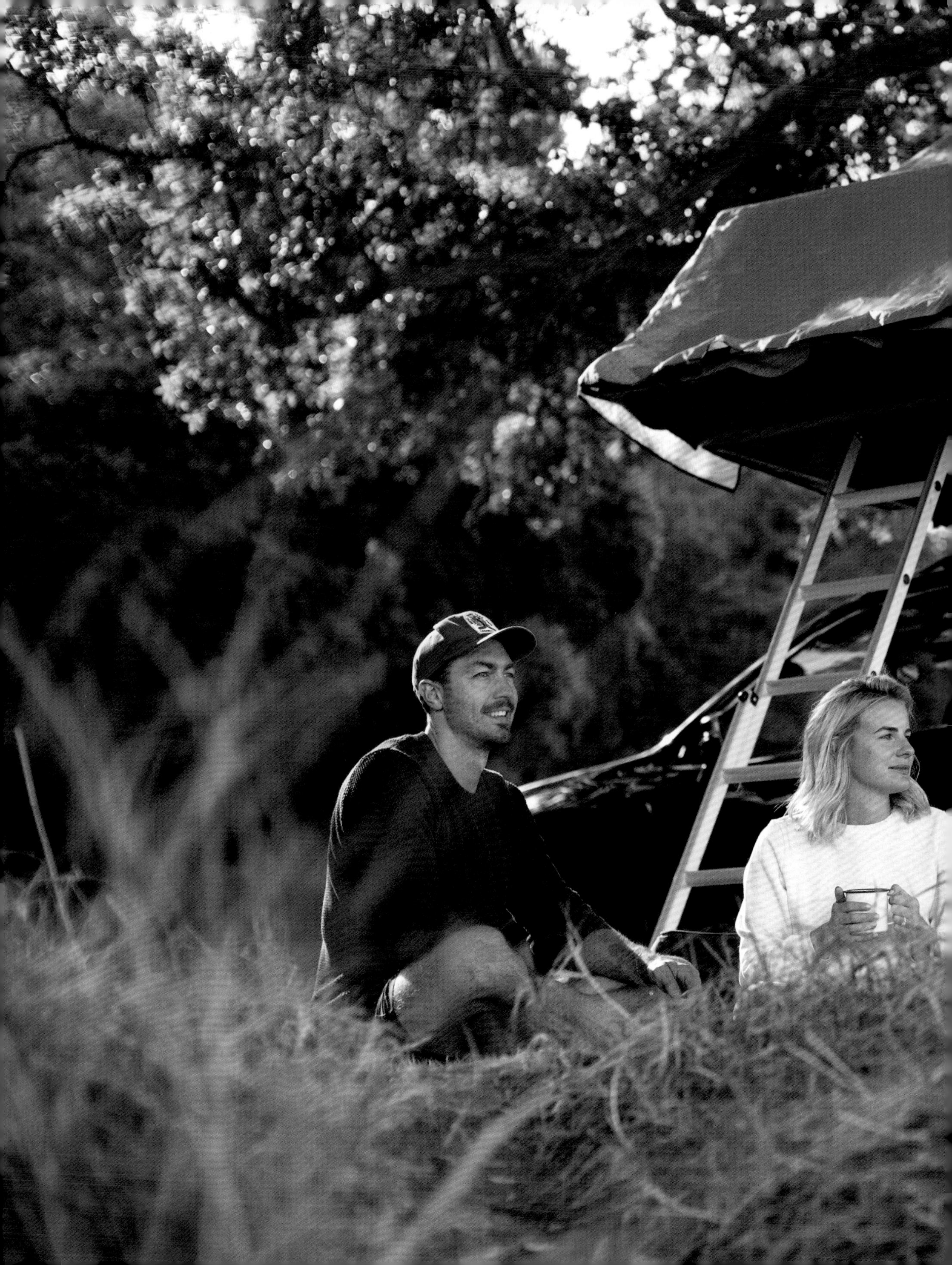

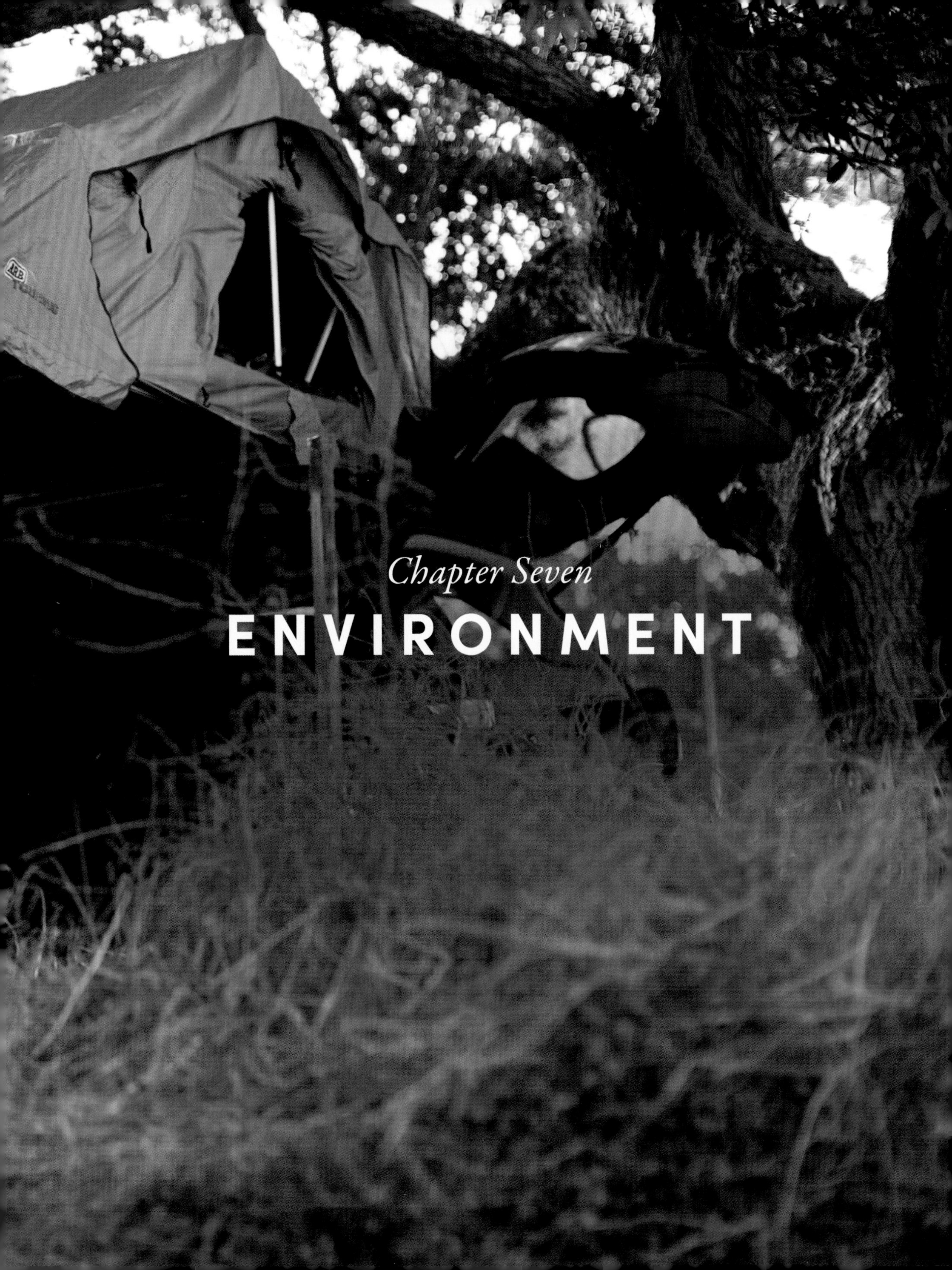

Chapter Seven

ENVIRONMENT

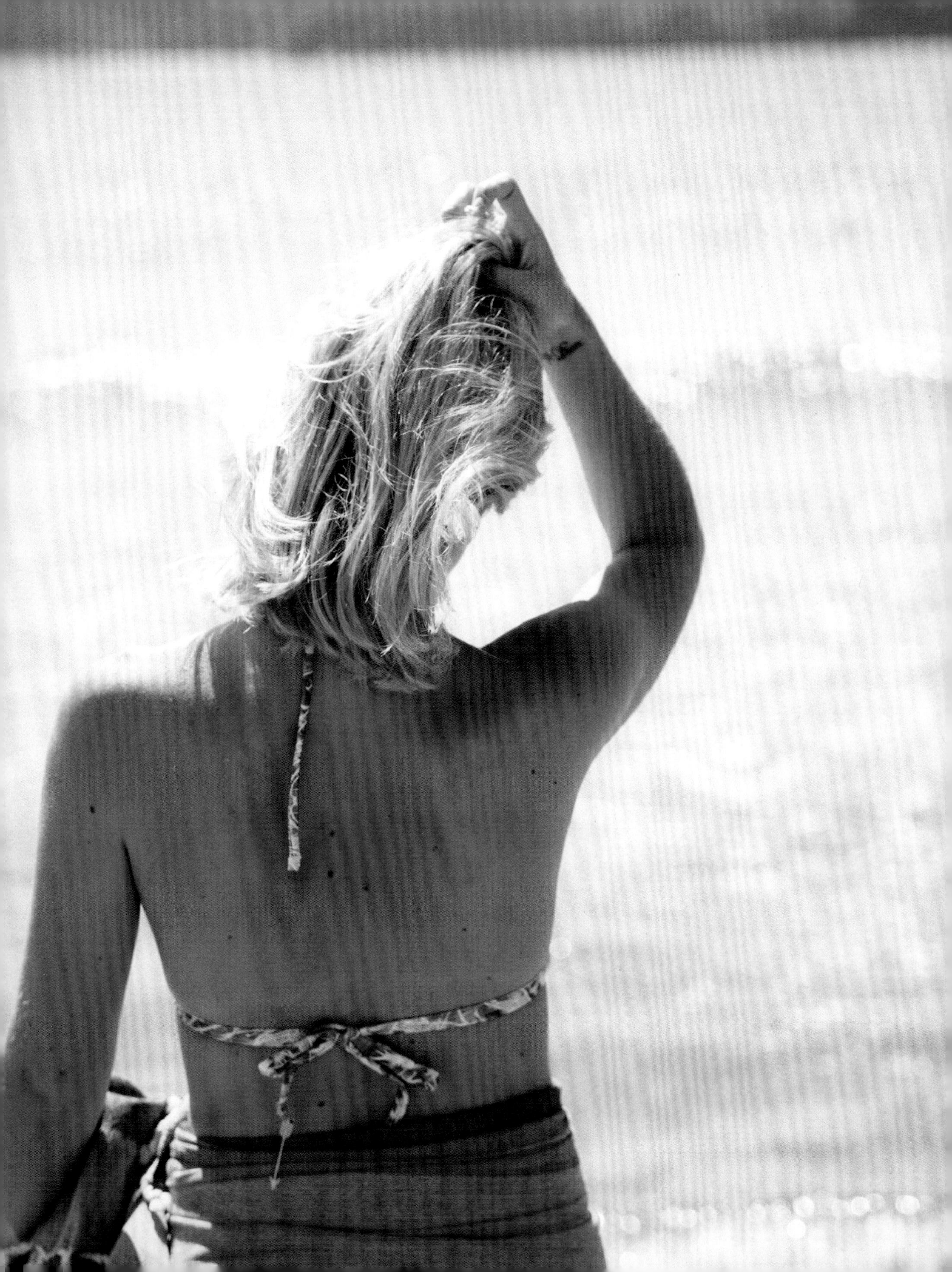

Now we've pretty well covered all the bits and bobs going on inside your body, but what about the stuff on the outside? What about the space you live in, and the things around you? What about the people you choose to have in your life? These things all have an effect on how you're feeling and your self-esteem too, so let's take a look at them.

I like to refer to all of these things as your 'environment'. When I talk about your 'environment', what I mean is essentially every single thing you choose to surround yourself with—your friends, your romantic partners, your workspace, your home and so on. Your environment has a huge impact upon how you're feeling, and on your actions and your thoughts, even if you don't realise it! If you fill your environment with positive, affirming and inspiring things then that naturally extends to how you feel about yourself and your life. There are some really simple things you can do right now to help your environment give you a boost, and I'm going to cover some of the things I've found most helpful in this chapter, so enjoy!

Also, I've used the word 'choose' deliberately there in my definition of what your environment is. I know that, in life, we don't always get to choose everything. We don't choose our family, as the saying goes, and sometimes we don't have much choice about the work we do to pay the bills. We don't choose the body we're born into, or who we fall in love with. However, even when our choices are a bit squished, I believe that we do still always have some things we can choose. Perhaps the only choice available to you at one time or another is to square your shoulders against the bad stuff and put a smile on your dial, but that's still a choice. You don't even have to believe in the smile—when it comes to smiling, sometimes all you have to do is fake it till you make it. In this sense, choice can be quite empowering, I think. Despite circumstances that might be less than ideal, you can still stand up for yourself and take the choices you do have in both hands.

So, with that in mind, the things you'll find in this chapter are just ideas. You don't have to go out and do everything I say. (You're the boss, not me!) Just do what works for you, and ignore the rest. And, maybe after reading this chapter, you might even come up with some of your own ideas for making your environment the best that it can possibly be. Whatever you do, I hope you'll soon start to see just how many positive side effects there are to making some changes in your environment. Have a go with some of the changes I suggest, and let me know how you feel.

YOUR SUPPORT CREW

Your self-esteem is strongly linked to the people you have around you. Have you ever had a terrible friendship or relationship where the other person is constantly negative, or subtly puts you down all the time? It starts to have a negative effect on your self-esteem, right?

Well, the good news is that the opposite is also true. When people are encouraging and loving, that has a positive effect on you too. That's why surrounding yourself with people who lift you up, make you laugh and bring out the best in you is key to leading a fulfilled life. Because happiness is contagious! People who know how to create their own happiness and who

When people are encouraging and loving, that has a positive effect on you too. That's why surrounding yourself with people who lift you up, make you laugh and bring out the best in you is key to leading a fulfilled life.

hand it around freely are the kinds of people you want in your life. A quote I always think of when it comes to relationships is this one often attributed to motivational speaker Jim Rohn: 'You are the average of the five people you spend the most time with.'

As I've said, you can't choose your family, but you can choose your friends—and, in lots of cases, your best friends can often become another kind of family! They're kind of like your hand-picked support crew: they cheer you on when you need it, believe in you when you might not believe in yourself, pick you up and dust you off when you fall, and give you their shoulder to cry on without judgement. At least, that's what they should be doing . . .

You can also choose your romantic partners, and it's actually really important that you do. If you're with someone who tells you you're not good enough, or puts you down, or makes you feel like an all-round crappy person, you need to get rid of that person *tout suite*. The same goes for your pals.

Sometimes, it can be difficult to see that a friend or partner isn't being very kind to you because you're caught in a trap of not being very kind to yourself. When you spend enough time with someone, you start to see the world through their eyes—and if, in their eyes, you never measure up, then it's not much of a surprise if you start feeling pretty rubbish about yourself. No one should ever make you feel like you aren't good enough. You *are* good enough. If someone in your life is making you feel anything less than awesome, it sounds like you might need to have a good hard look at whether you should be spending your precious time with that person. In my experience, this is where good friends or trusted family members are worth their weight in gold—often, they're the ones who can see that someone isn't being nice to you, and will point it out. If your friends or family are telling you this, it's worth at least hearing them out.

If you're anything like me, you might find yourself picking up the mannerisms of the people you spend the most time with. Sound familiar? It's quite an odd phenomenon, but I notice it in myself all the time. A while back, I read about a 2014 study conducted by University of Colorado Boulder that

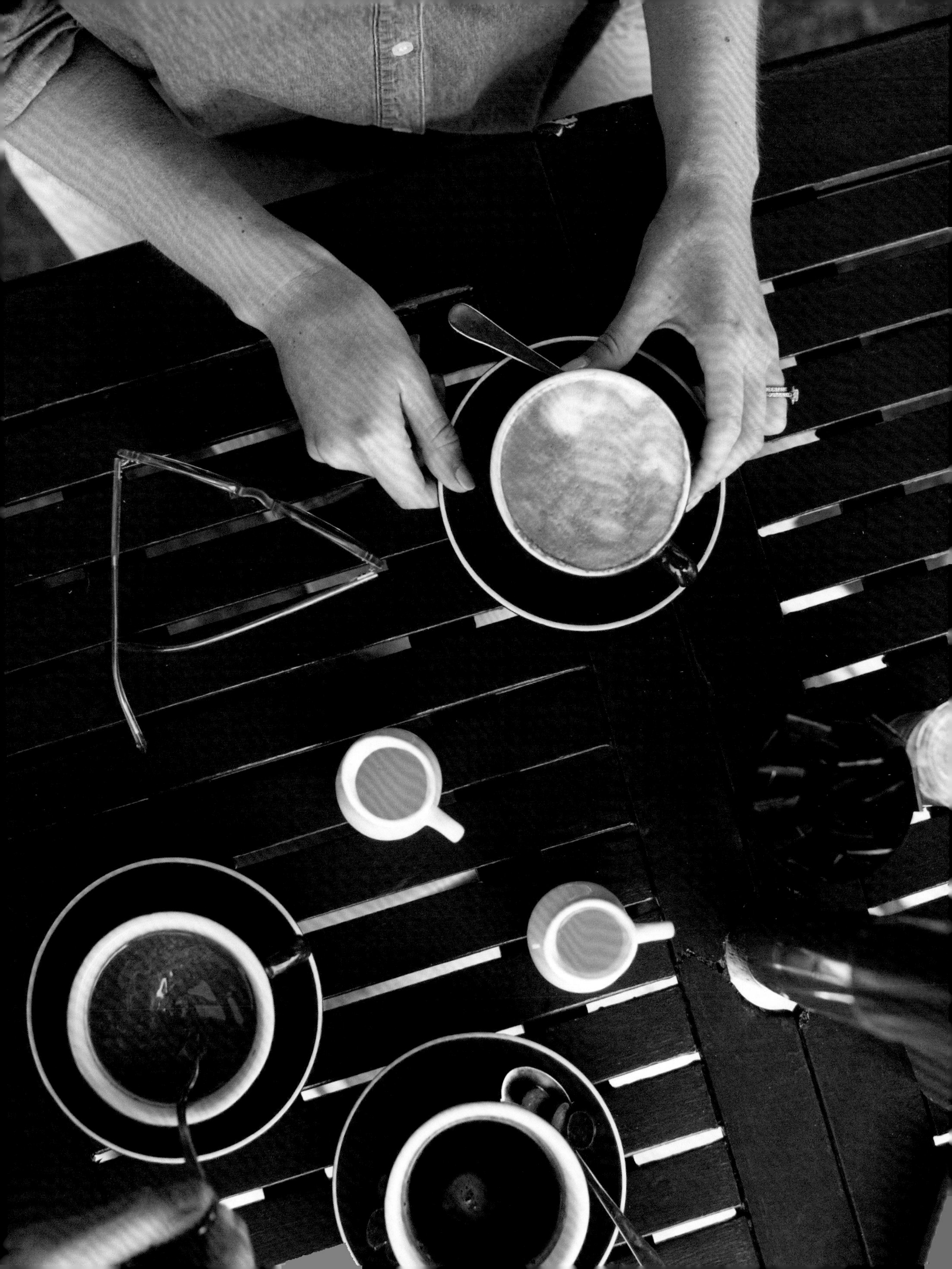

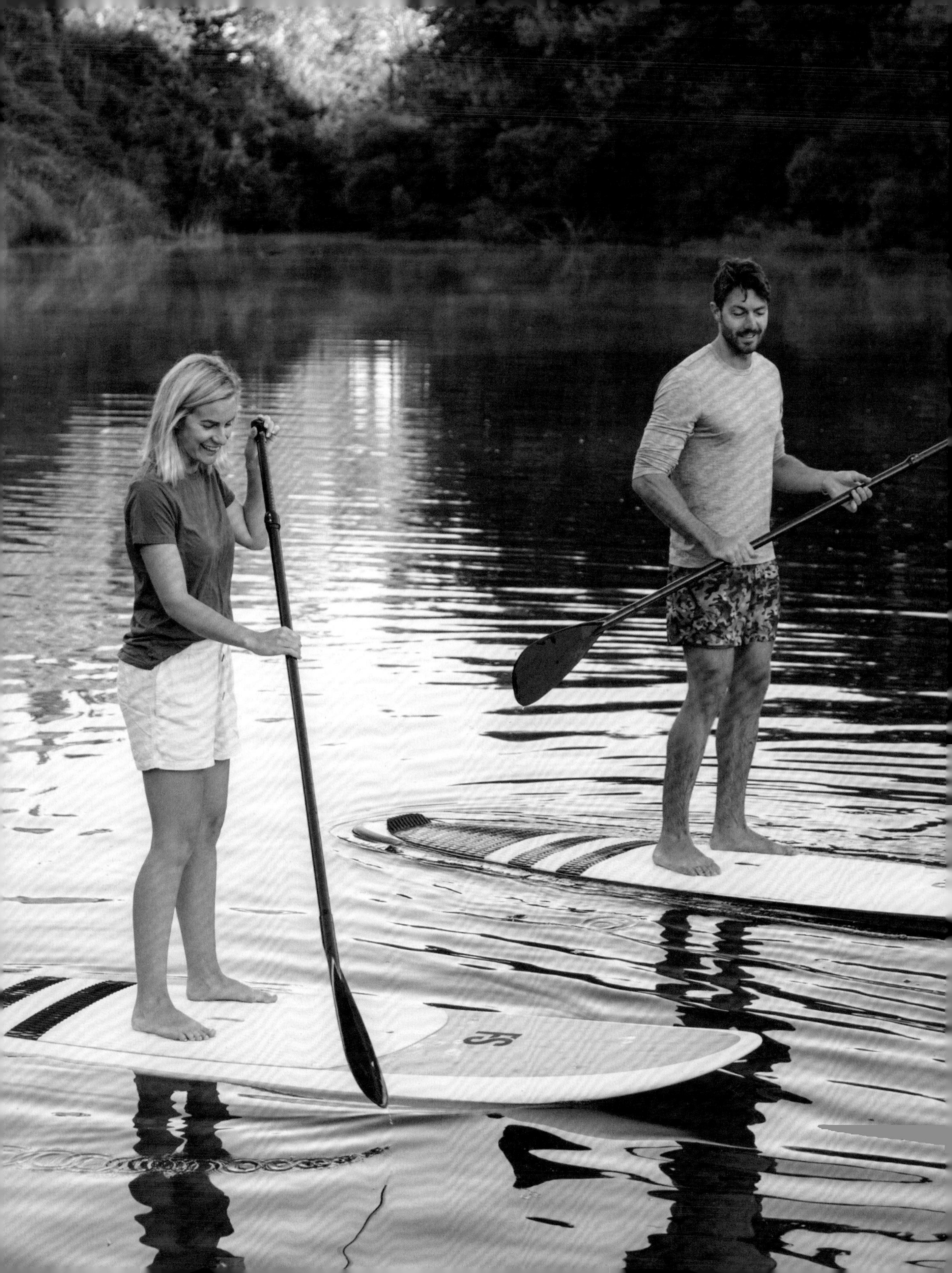

suggested we tend to go for long-term partners who have similar DNA to us. This made me wonder if the same goes for our friends. Maybe we pick people who are so similar to us that it's easy to adopt their mannerisms? Bit of a tangent, I admit, but it's an interesting thought.

There is also some really interesting research out there that suggests that strong relationships contribute to a long, healthy and happy life. I think, as human beings, we need social interaction on whatever level. For many of us, social media has slowly come to replace either some or a lot of our face-to-face social interactions with an online version, which is very different and nowhere near as satisfying. It's important to make an effort to see your friends and loved ones in real life when you can—chatting to them in comment threads on social media isn't the same thing as a good old in-person conversation.

It's important to find people who you enjoy spending time with. Now, I'm not talking about becoming a full-on extrovert if you're not naturally that way inclined. While some of us love attention and feed off being surrounded by heaps of people, others of us find constant people contact exhausting and instead prefer a quieter life with just a few really close friends (some of whom might be cats—cough, I am that person, cough). Personally, I prefer a good mixture of both. I think I am some sort of 'extroverted introvert'. I love being around people sometimes, but I also crave alone time after a while and will cancel plans if I feel like being by myself. Wherever you fall on the extrovert–introvert scale, it's cool! And it's especially cool to know yourself well enough to understand how much people contact is enough for you. But the fact still stands that all of us—introverts and extroverts alike—need friends. We all love to be loved, am I right?

I know that making friends isn't always easy. In fact, sometimes the experience can be hard and frankly disheartening. You might meet someone who you think is the bee's knees . . . but maybe they're not as keen on the friendship as you are. Or you might know a few people who hang out together and have known each other for ages, but whenever you're with them you feel like the awkward newbie imposter. These feelings are super normal—and, even though they can be really isolating, it can help to remember that lots of us have them! Even when you feel alone, you're not really alone. There's probably someone you know who feels exactly the same way, but you just don't know it yet. That's why it's important to reach out to others—and to keep reaching out, even when you feel like it's not doing anything. You never know the ripple effects of your actions.

I moved to Melbourne when I was nineteen, and when I got there I didn't know a soul. I moved in with two lovely Kiwi girls, and that gave me some sense of home, but I still found it really difficult to make friends. I tried to use that time positively, by getting to know myself better and trying to be more comfortable in my own company. At the same time, I also balanced it out with a healthy dose of getting out of my comfort zone in order to meet people—which I did, eventually! It just took time, and it was definitely worth it in the end.

If you're wondering about how, exactly, you might start searching out some new friendships, I've included a couple of tips in the action plan opposite for you, along with some other tips about your support crew in general.

WORKSPACE WELL-BEING

Your workspace is another incredibly important environment for your well-being. If you're stuck in a job you hate, and you're slogging it out to get a promotion or a pay rise, or just because it will 'look good on your CV', then don't. Life is far too precious to be working in a shitty job, and times have changed since the days of having to stay in the same job for 40 years. It's much more acceptable now to move around jobs until you find the right one for you. Put the feelers out, and start making some changes. Because, after all, your life is in your control and yours only!

That said, you might simply need to make the choice to change your

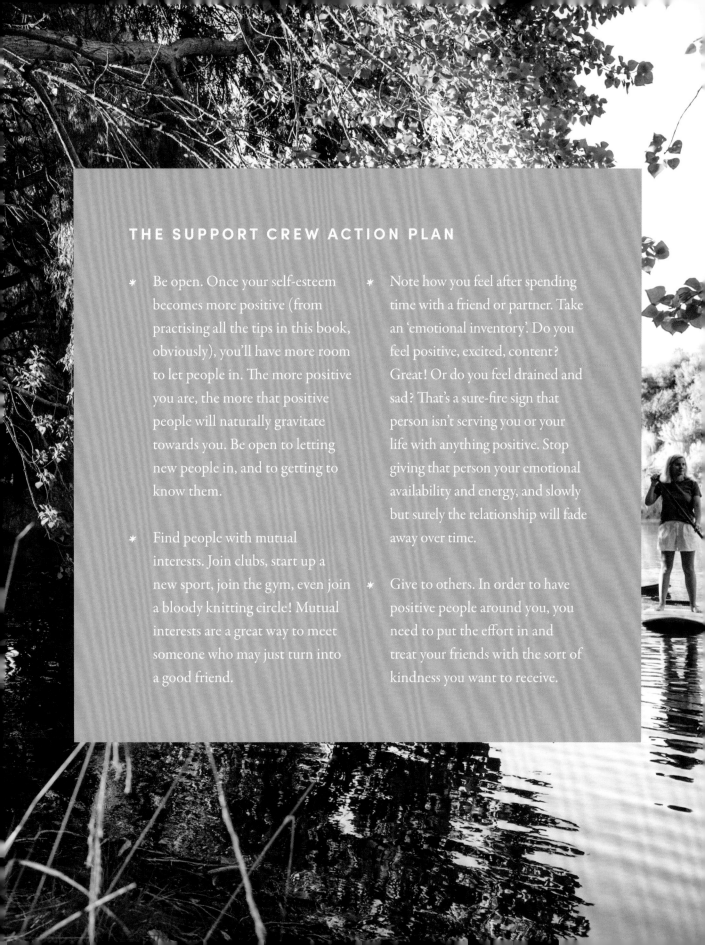

THE SUPPORT CREW ACTION PLAN

✳ Be open. Once your self-esteem becomes more positive (from practising all the tips in this book, obviously), you'll have more room to let people in. The more positive you are, the more that positive people will naturally gravitate towards you. Be open to letting new people in, and to getting to know them.

✳ Find people with mutual interests. Join clubs, start up a new sport, join the gym, even join a bloody knitting circle! Mutual interests are a great way to meet someone who may just turn into a good friend.

✳ Note how you feel after spending time with a friend or partner. Take an 'emotional inventory'. Do you feel positive, excited, content? Great! Or do you feel drained and sad? That's a sure-fire sign that person isn't serving you or your life with anything positive. Stop giving that person your emotional availability and energy, and slowly but surely the relationship will fade away over time.

✳ Give to others. In order to have positive people around you, you need to put the effort in and treat your friends with the sort of kindness you want to receive.

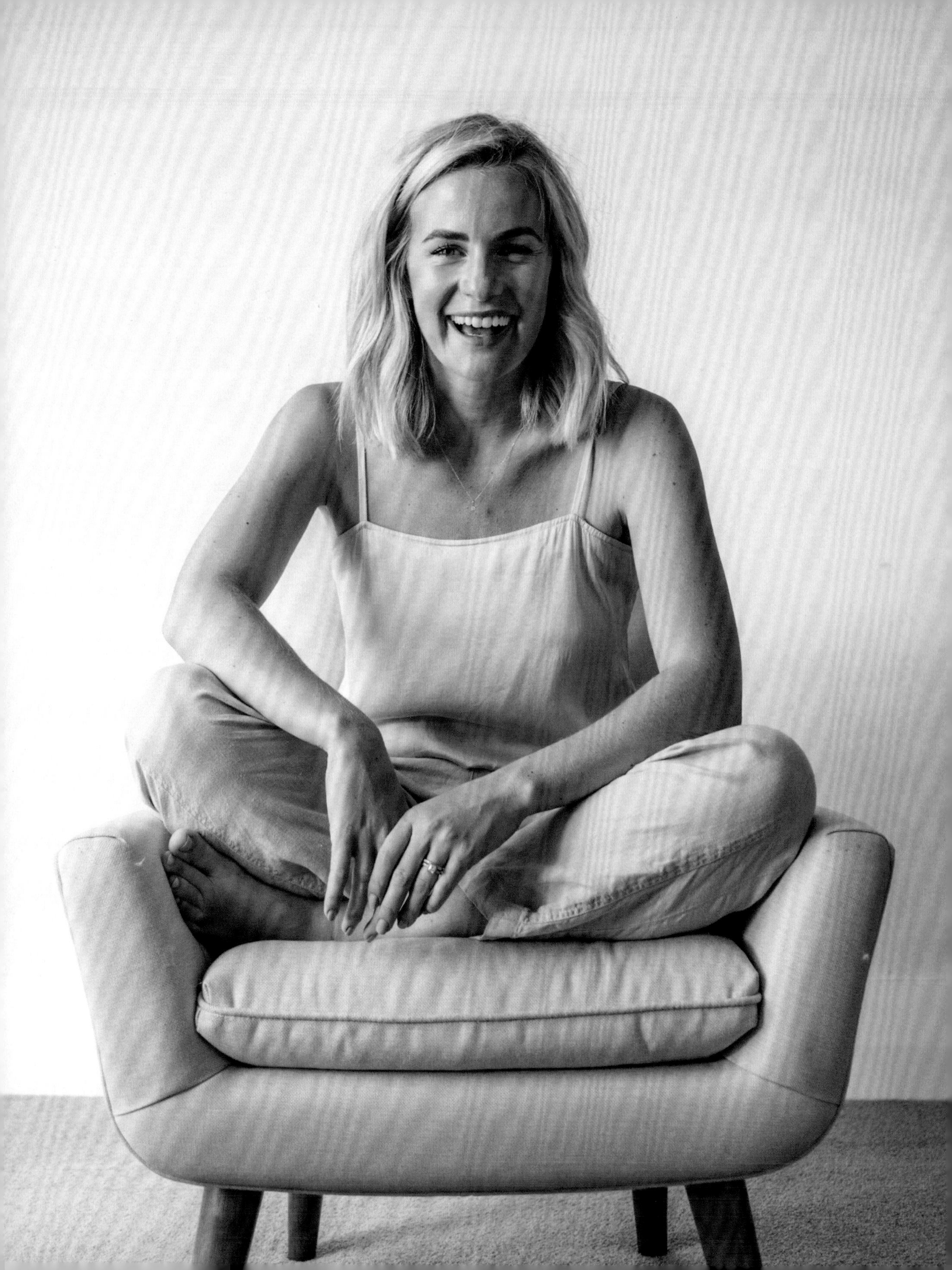

perspective on your job. A lot of people think their job sucks, when it might not actually be that bad—they hate it simply because they keep telling themselves they hate it. If they wanted to take the glass-half-full approach, they could see it as a means to an end. When you get paid to do a job, you can then use that money for all sorts of needs and wants in your life. Also, in many ways, having a job you get paid for is a HUGE privilege, especially if you are getting paid fairly. There are an awful lot of people in this world who don't get paid for their hard work (like stay-at-home mothers and caregivers, for example), so it can be worthwhile taking an honest look at your job and working out whether it does actually suck—or if it's potentially your attitude that sucks.

Here are some questions you can ask yourself to see your job for what it really is.

* Do I get paid fairly for my time, and do I get time off that I can use to do whatever I want?

* Do I earn enough money that I can afford nice food, rent, and maybe even cool things like holidays or eating out?

* Do I have supportive and fun colleagues who I enjoy spending the work hours with?

* Does my boss (if you have one) respect and understand me and my ambitions?

* Is there scope for me to advance if I want to? Can I aim for a promotion, or can I ask for extra training that'll give me skills I don't currently have?

If most of your answers to the above questions were 'yes', then perhaps your job isn't as bad as it seems. Of course, if you hate your job for very good reasons—such as being overworked, underpaid and treated badly by your colleagues or managers, or you're just plain bored to tears—then you definitely need to make some moves in a different direction.

When you feel good about the work you're doing, you tend to feel good about yourself. It's pretty likely that you might spend more time at work than you do with your friends and family, so it's important that it's a positive experience, one that is 'filling your cup' in one way or another. A great way to do this is to celebrate your wins. If you've had a good review, or landed a new client, or even just had a positive interaction with someone, give yourself a little reward. It doesn't have to be tangible; it can just be a simple pause-and-reflect moment. Or it could be an afternoon hot chocolate. You decide!

Another great way to boost your self-esteem through your work environment is to realise the effect your work has on those around you. Instead of doing it for yourself, think about them. Maybe it's your co-workers, who will really appreciate a thorough job from you because it makes their day a little easier. Or, if you're working in hospitality, think of how your demeanour and energy can impact someone else's day. It's great to remember that when you do things to help others, it not only helps them but it usually helps you too.

No matter where you work—whether it's in an office or for yourself at home—creating a positive environment can make an enormous difference to your happiness and productivity levels. These days, I mostly work from home, and I find that if I have clutter in my office that translates to clutter in my mind. Transitioning to working at home actually forced me to take a closer look at the things that were helping keep me motivated at work, and the things that weren't. I had to figure out some useful habits to help get me in the work mindset. The bonus is that I think these habits apply to any workspace anywhere! So I've included the tips and tricks that have worked for me in the workspace action plan over the page, and they might just do wonders for your workspace too.

No matter where you work—
whether it's in an office or for
yourself at home—setting a
positive environment can make
an enormous difference to your
happiness and productivity levels.

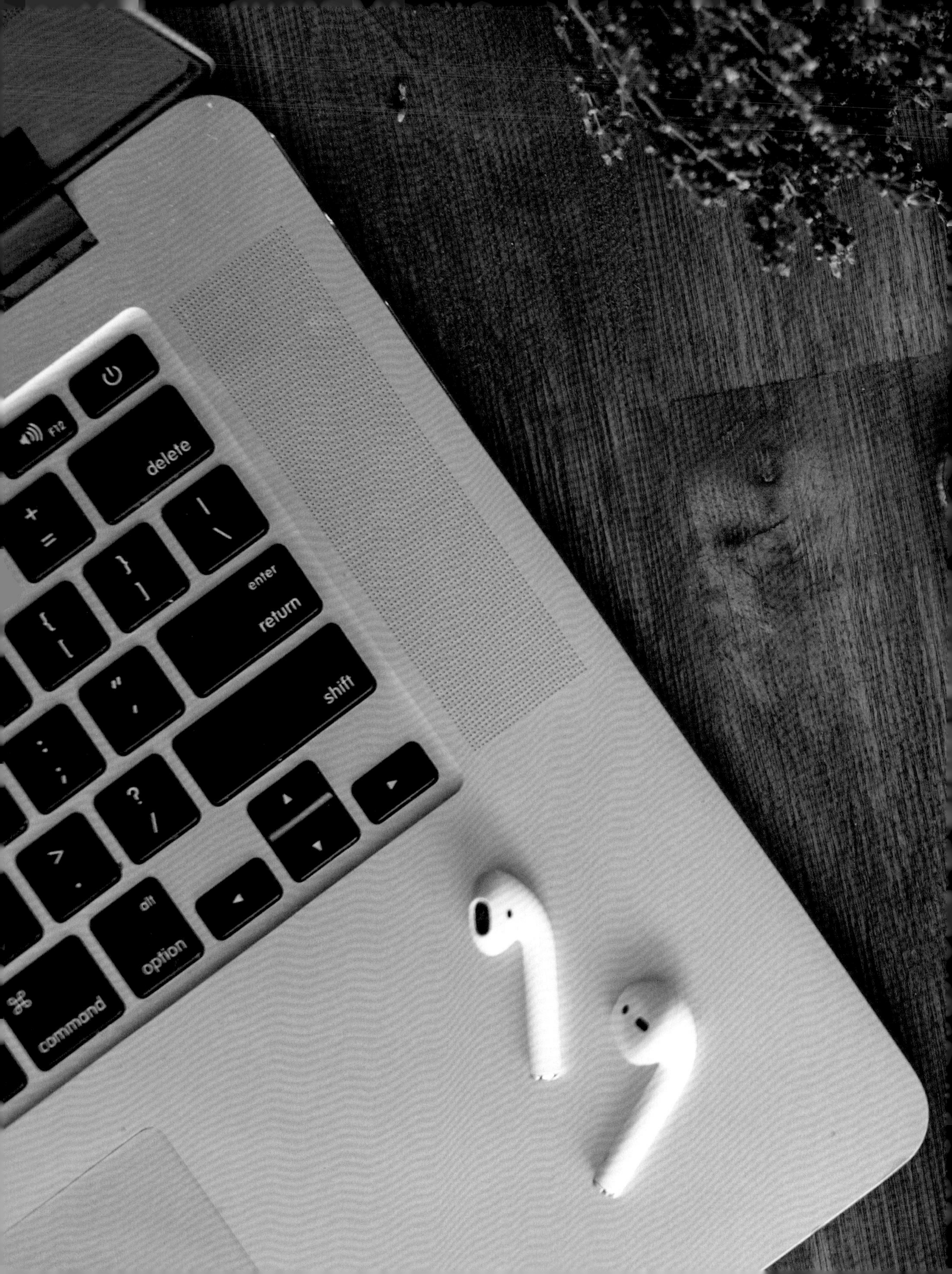
F12
delete
enter
return
shift
alt
option
command

THE WORKSPACE ACTION PLAN

* Wake up early, and get ready for work. If you work at home, treat your home office with the same respect you would any other office. Get up, have a shower and get dressed in something smart. This is a great way to trick your mind into 'get stuff done' mode. I find that if I start working in my dressing gown or trackies (which can happen—I'm not perfect), it can be a slippery slope. I try to get back into my work routine asap.

* Have a clear desk. It took me ages to figure out a good storage system at home. This is something that I suddenly realised was actually a bit of admin when I had to work it out myself, but it was so worth it. Now, I know where things go and I've got a good system set up, and it just takes a whole layer of stress away. Far preferable to having bits of paper everywhere and a whole mess that turns into an abyss where all the important things go and never return from!

* Get rid of distractions. When you have something important to do, close your email and focus. (I promise it won't be the end of the world if you don't reply to every single email immediately . . . Unless you have a job that is life-and-death related. Then maybe keep your emails open.) If I REALLY need to focus on something, I put my phone in another room. However, if you're worried about missing important calls, there are some really great apps that will block social media for you. My favourite is Offtime (offtime.app), which lets you choose which apps to block for a while; you can even block calls and texts, if you're that way inclined. I find it really helpful if I don't trust myself not to get distracted by the constant call of my Instagram DMs.

>>

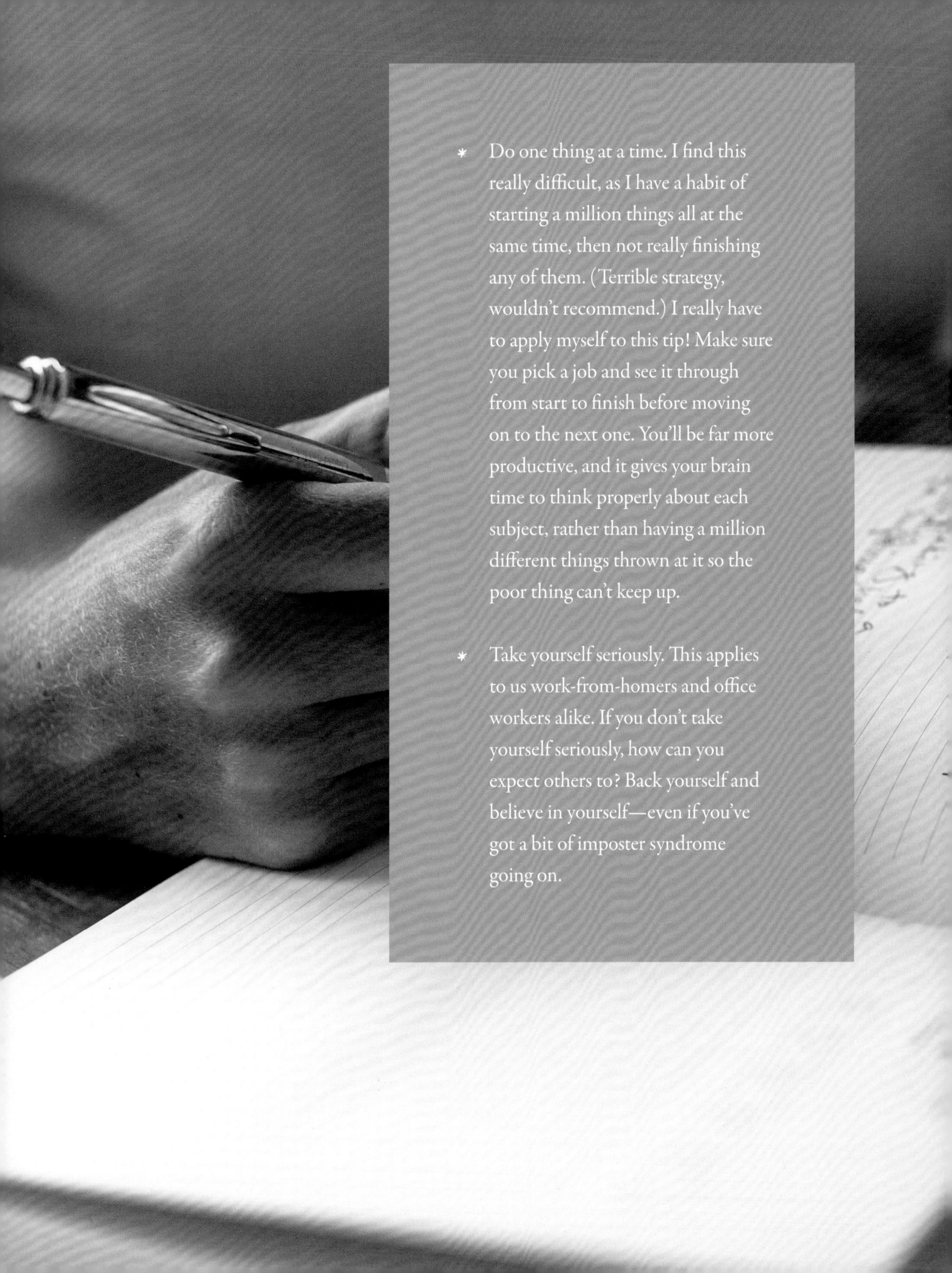

* Do one thing at a time. I find this really difficult, as I have a habit of starting a million things all at the same time, then not really finishing any of them. (Terrible strategy, wouldn't recommend.) I really have to apply myself to this tip! Make sure you pick a job and see it through from start to finish before moving on to the next one. You'll be far more productive, and it gives your brain time to think properly about each subject, rather than having a million different things thrown at it so the poor thing can't keep up.

* Take yourself seriously. This applies to us work-from-homers and office workers alike. If you don't take yourself seriously, how can you expect others to? Back yourself and believe in yourself—even if you've got a bit of imposter syndrome going on.

* If you work at home, try to have a separate area to do your work. For so long I persevered with the dining table as my office, and thought it was fine—but the reality was that I found it difficult to stop myself from getting distracted because it didn't feel 'different' enough to normal home life. I would suddenly be cleaning the pantry at 10 a.m. on a Wednesday, or constantly making toast. It's amazing how much toast one can eat when one is avoiding working on something. Now, I have a small home office, and find it really beneficial to my productivity levels.

* Take breaks. It's important to get outside for some fresh air every now and then. If you're feeling a little frustrated or overwhelmed, go for a walk around the block, or eat your lunch outside. It's amazing what fresh air can do.

* Get nice stationery. I know it sounds a bit silly, but having nice matching stationery gives me motivation to keep my desk organised and clear. Maybe it's the effect Pinterest has had on me (I think that's the most basic thing I've ever said), but I get really satisfied when everything is nice and neat and has pretty colours. It doesn't have to be expensive, but if it gives you motivation then it's worth doing.

* Respect your own time. Don't work all hours of the day and night to impress the people you work with at the expense of your happiness. Schedule in time for leisure activities and try to avoid letting work bleed in to your off time—unless it's totally unavoidable (which, let's be honest, does happen!). Letting work take over can lead to you resenting the work, which isn't helpful for anyone.

HOME SWEET HOME

Don't think I've forgotten about your home life! Your home environment is just as important (actually more, in my humble opinion) as your work environment for your overall well-being. It's important to have a space that feels like it represents you, and a place you can be proud of. It doesn't matter whether it's big or small, and whether or not it's your own home or a place you rent or share with your family. There are so many small changes that can make your home life feel comfortable, and more 'you'.

Having a space to call home, where you feel comfortable and like you can totally be yourself, can really positively contribute to how you feel about yourself. In my experience, I've found that showing a bit of pride in my home and putting in a bit of effort actually encourages me to do the same in other aspects of my life. And it's as easy as starting with a clean bedroom.

THE HOME ACTION PLAN

* Make your bed. It's kind of hilarious how simple this is. If you're anything like me, you grew up with your parents telling you to do this every day and you never listened! Gretchen Rubin, author of *The Happiness Project*, explains that this three-minute task is one of the simplest habits you can adopt to positively impact your happiness. It puts your brain into 'task mode' and gives you some positive satisfaction, because you've already ticked off one thing on your to-do list—so you're ready for the next!

* Invest in things that bring experience. Instead of buying cushions, go for things like a fondue set, or a pizza stone for your oven. These things will encourage you to have people over and therefore increase that beautiful human connection I keep banging on about. I mean, cushions are great too, but you get where I'm going with this, right?

* Keep your bedroom tidy. My bedroom is just like my work environment, in that I feel so much clearer in my mind when everything is put away. I feel like I sleep better too. A great way to keep on top of it is to make sure you have a good system going. For example, make sure you have specific spaces for specific items. I can always tell things are starting to get away on me in life when my bedroom gets messy. The two go completely hand in hand.

* Get some green in your home. I am obsessed with plants, even though I can't keep them alive to save myself—but I try! They bring so much happiness and calmness to my home. And they don't just look delightful; they also actually help to purify the air and can even raise the air's humidity. Some of my favourite air-purifying plants are spider plants, aloe vera, snake plants, chrysanthemums, peace lilies and bamboo palms.

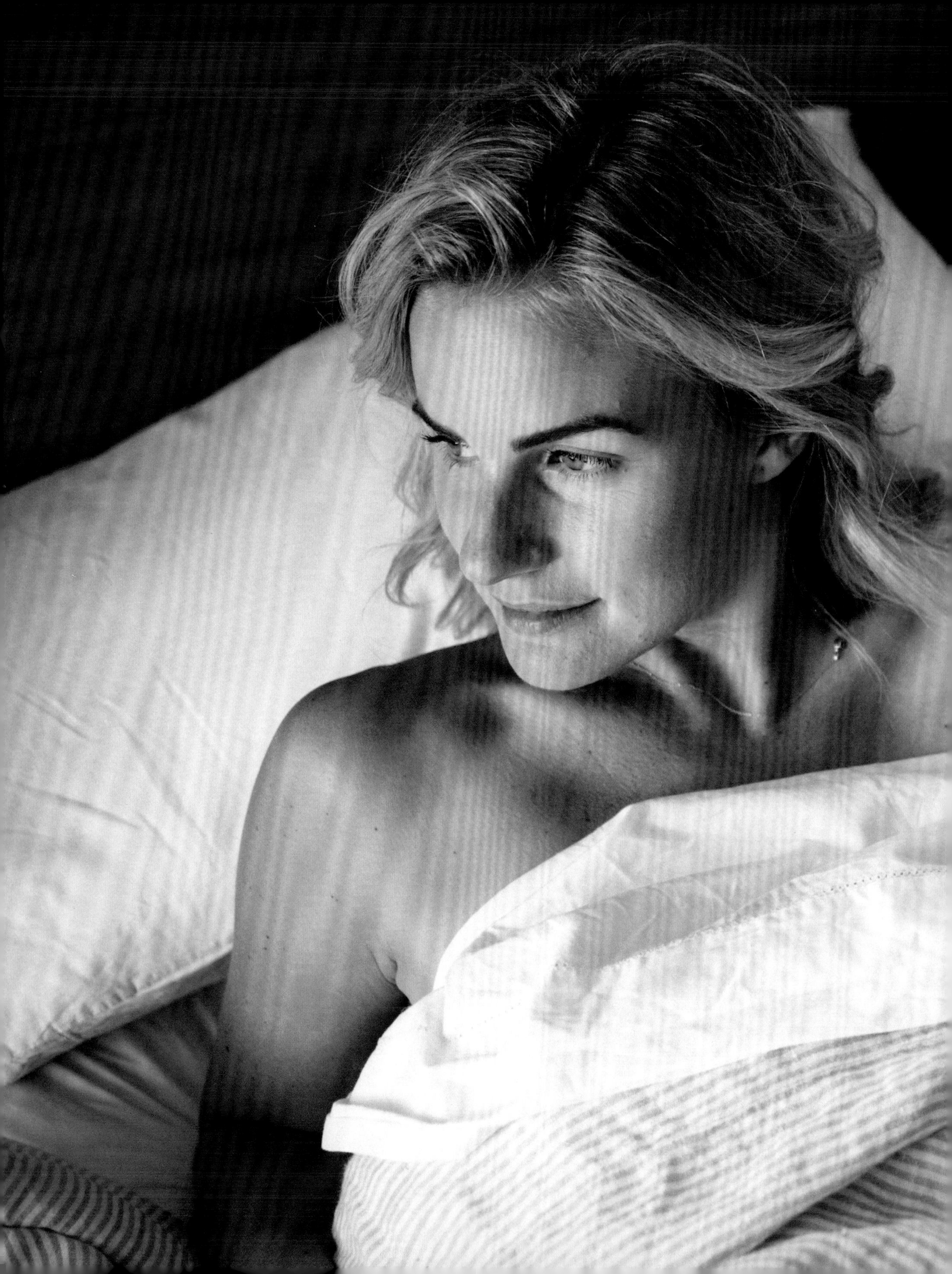

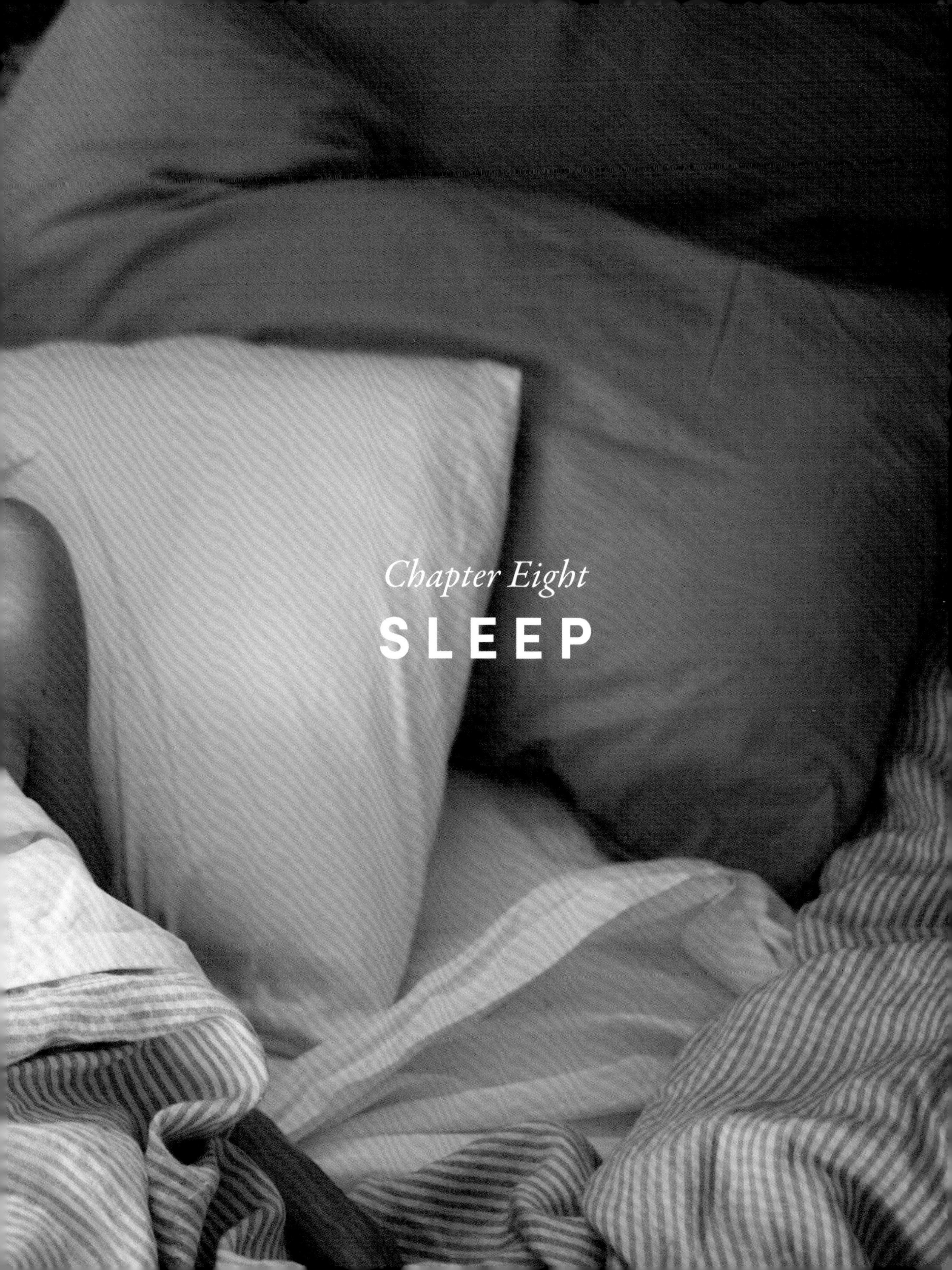

Chapter Eight

SLEEP

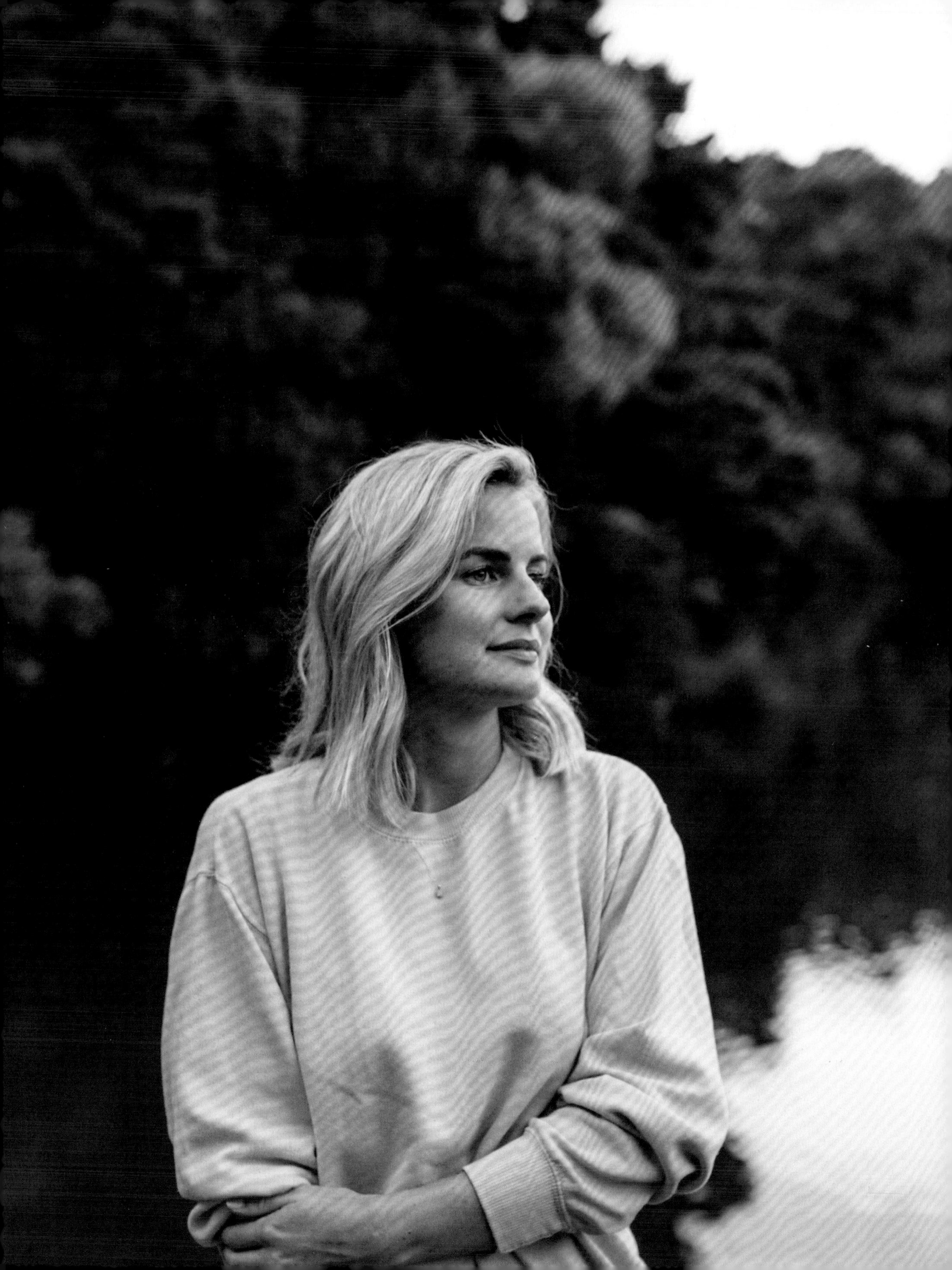

There's a lot of discussion out there about what defines success. Once upon a time, people thought that how busy you were related directly to how important you were. It was like a badge of honour to be super-duper busy. Thankfully, over recent years we've started to see this idea dismantled. We've moved away from 'glorifying busy' and towards the idea that it's a better idea to work smarter, not harder. And, you know what goes along with this idea of not putting so much emphasis on busy-ness? Making sure you give yourself time for rest, and more specifically sleep.

I have to say that this shift has been music to my ears! When I was growing up, I remember hearing stories about how the most successful leaders in the world only got around four or five hours of sleep a night, and that the only way to climb the corporate ladder was to work 80 hours a week. It's refreshing (and a relief!) to see that view shifting. It's no longer all about who is in the office the longest or 'whoever gets the least amount of sleep is obviously the hardest worker'. Now, it's more about taking the time to look after yourself, so that the work you do is of a higher quality and not necessarily just a higher quantity.

And sleep isn't just important on the work front. It's a massive aspect of your all-round health and well-being. When your self-esteem is flagging, sometimes the only boost it needs is a good night's sleep. Getting a decent sleep can help to refresh your body and your mind so that you wake up feeling stronger and better equipped to deal with the peaks and pitfalls of the day to come. Of course, sometimes it's more than sleep that you need, but I do find that a good sleep can do wonders in terms of helping me to feel a bit more on top of things than I did the day before.

I know that you can't always control your sleep hours—I'm looking at you, parents of small children—but when you can, it's worth taking it seriously. The good news is that, even if you are living with a tiny sleep-thief, there are still some tricks and tips you can put to use to prioritise getting a good sleep when you're able to.

WHY SLEEP MATTERS

We live in a world where it can sometimes feel like we have to be 'on' all the time. This is probably thanks, at least in part, to social media, where people can portray whatever kind of life they like. (Whether they actually live that life is another story . . .) We are constantly comparing our own personal busy-ness with a potentially false standard of 'busy' that other people present on social media. What's more, the introduction of smart phones (which have become an extension of the human arm) has led to a pretty common expectation that everyone should be contactable all the time. It can feel impossible to escape and get some time out to switch off.

In response, lots of us go ahead and make ourselves so busy that we don't ever have any time to stop and rest—and, not surprisingly, just end up feeling panicky and anxious. Sound familiar? Maybe you're a chronic overcommitter (guilty as charged), afraid to ever say no and full of FOMO. The price of all this busy-ness, of course, is your sleep. When you get way too busy—and I mean both in real terms and also just in your head—it's your sleep time that often takes the hit.

Getting a decent sleep can
help to refresh your body and
your mind so that you wake
up feeling stronger and better
equipped to deal with the peaks
and pitfalls of the day to come.

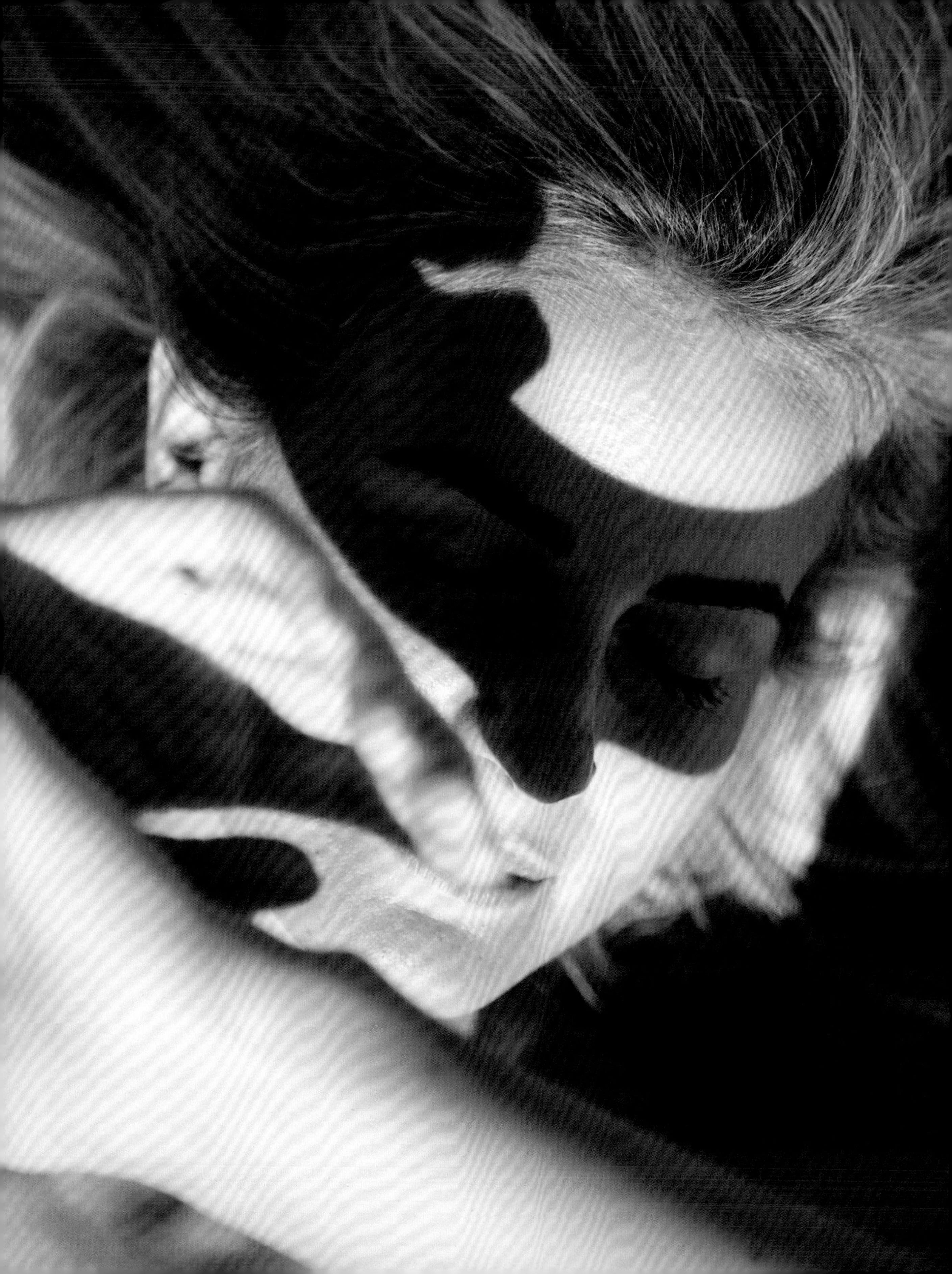

I've always been quite a good sleeper (one of those 'could sleep through a brass band' types), but when my anxiety was at an all-time high while I was living in London my sleep took a massive nosedive. It would take me *hours* just to get to sleep, then I'd wake up multiple times during the night and be wide awake all over again at a ridiculously early hour. Honestly, I felt like I was going crazy. It was awful. I found it difficult to concentrate at work, and I was extremely irritable and very sensitive. I was constantly upset about something—usually really small things that wouldn't bother me at all now. It really did suck. I'm sure those of you who struggle with anxiety or battle with getting to sleep know the feeling. It's not nice.

Sleep is really, really important for your mental health and your self-esteem. It's so important that we should all be making it a number-one priority. When you get enough sleep, it can make everything feel so much more manageable! You don't feel as depressed, anxious or edgy, and you do feel better prepared to face the day ahead. You find it easier to make good decisions about things like what you eat and how you handle stressful situations.

Don't believe me? Well then, here's some science.

THE SCIENCE OF SLEEP

Back in the old days—like, *long* before you or I were around—people used to live by the sun. They would get up with the sun and go to bed with the sun. Then, along came electricity and the ability to have light after dark. Now, we can stay up as long as we like! (And I do tend to faff around a lot at bedtime myself—much to Art's annoyance.) However, as wonderful as artificial light at night can be, it's not so wonderful in the sense that, if you let it, it can really mess with your circadian rhythm.

We all have a circadian rhythm. It's basically a 24-hour internal clock that runs in the background of your brain and cycles between sleepiness and

As well as helping to regulate your circadian rhythm, there's a whole bunch of other benefits to sleep in terms of your well-being.

alertness at regular intervals. It's also known as your sleep–wake cycle. An out-of-whack circadian rhythm can affect your sleep, but it's also been linked to a bunch of diseases, including cancer, diabetes, heart disease and obesity. Scary.

As well as helping to regulate your circadian rhythm, there's a whole bunch of other benefits to sleep in terms of your well-being. In fact, a good night's sleep has so many benefits that I don't even know where to begin—but I've had a crack, and compiled this list for your reading pleasure. (I do love a good list.)

* **It makes your brain work.** Brain performance is kind of a biggie, right? Well, according to the National Sleep Foundation in the US (sleepfoundation.org), people who have longer hours of more restful sleep have been shown to form better short-term and long-term memories, have faster reaction times AND are better at performing more difficult mental tasks. I don't know about you, but that all sounds pretty good to me!

* **It's great for your health.** Not getting enough sleep every night can actually have a negative impact on your immune system, leaving you more likely to get sick. And here's where it gets a bit scary—a study from Harvard Medical School in 2007 found that not getting enough sleep could also increase your risk of heart disease and diabetes. Yikes. What's more, not getting enough sleep just makes you tired (obviously), which can make you crave energy-dense food that's not that great for your health—3 p. m. sugar fix, anyone?

* **You can be an athlete!** OK, it might not turn you into LeBron James (it's not a miracle worker), but getting enough sleep can improve your athletic performance. For instance, one University

of Pittsburgh study looked at over 2800 women and found that poor sleep was linked to slower walking, lower grip strength and greater difficulty performing independent activities.

* **It makes you feel good.** As I've mentioned, sleep has a massive impact on your mental well-being and, as a result, how you feel about yourself.

We are finding out more and more every day about how a lack of sleep can have a poor effect on our mental and physical health, and on our self-esteem. (Again, when I say 'we' here, I mean 'scientists'.) If you've ever had a bad night's sleep, you will know how it can send your irritability through the roof. A thing that wouldn't usually bother you can become the most annoying thing in the entire world. Maybe your partner is eating just that little bit too loudly, or your sleeve gets caught on a door handle, flinging you backwards. These things tend not to bother us if we're feeling good, but sleep-deprived us is a little more on the titchy side. Also, you can find yourself feeling really easily overwhelmed by things, and your emotional barriers can become almost non-existent. Of course, this all just leads to even more stress.

Sleep deprivation has also been shown to increase your sensitivity. It can mean you take things more personally than you otherwise might, and this leads to feelings of fear, frustration and self-doubt. Maybe someone says, 'You look nice today', and instead of simply saying, 'Oh, thank you', you say, 'Oh, so I usually look TERRIBLE, DO I, SHARON?'—a classic example of sensitivity. In this way, a lack of sleep can be a real challenge to relationships with friends or family. When little things are getting to you more than they need to, it can feel as though things are a far bigger deal than they really are. You can find yourself feeling unhappy with yourself and with your loved ones, and that can be a huge blow to everyone's confidence, not just yours.

One interesting study from the University of California, Berkeley, looked at

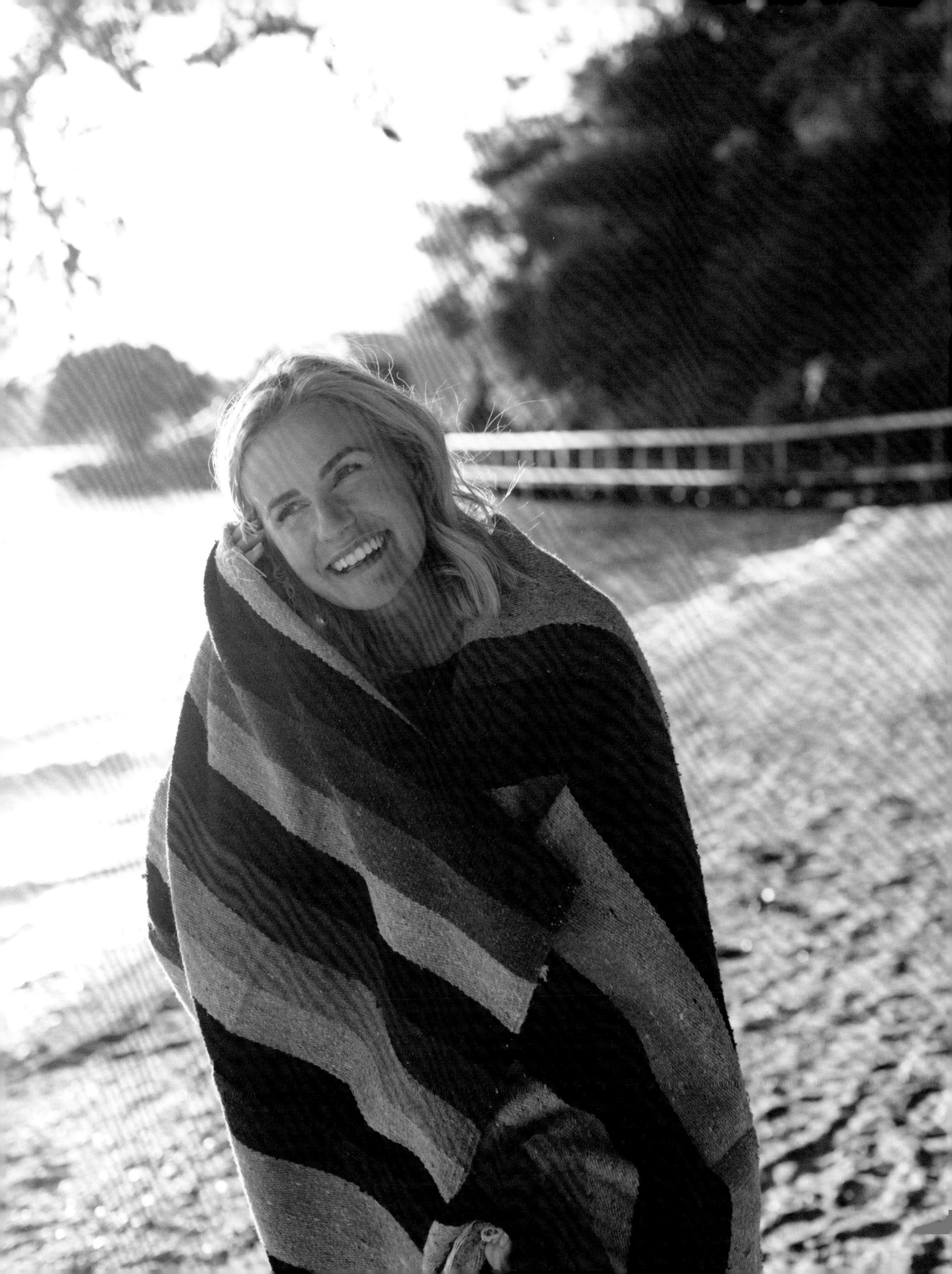

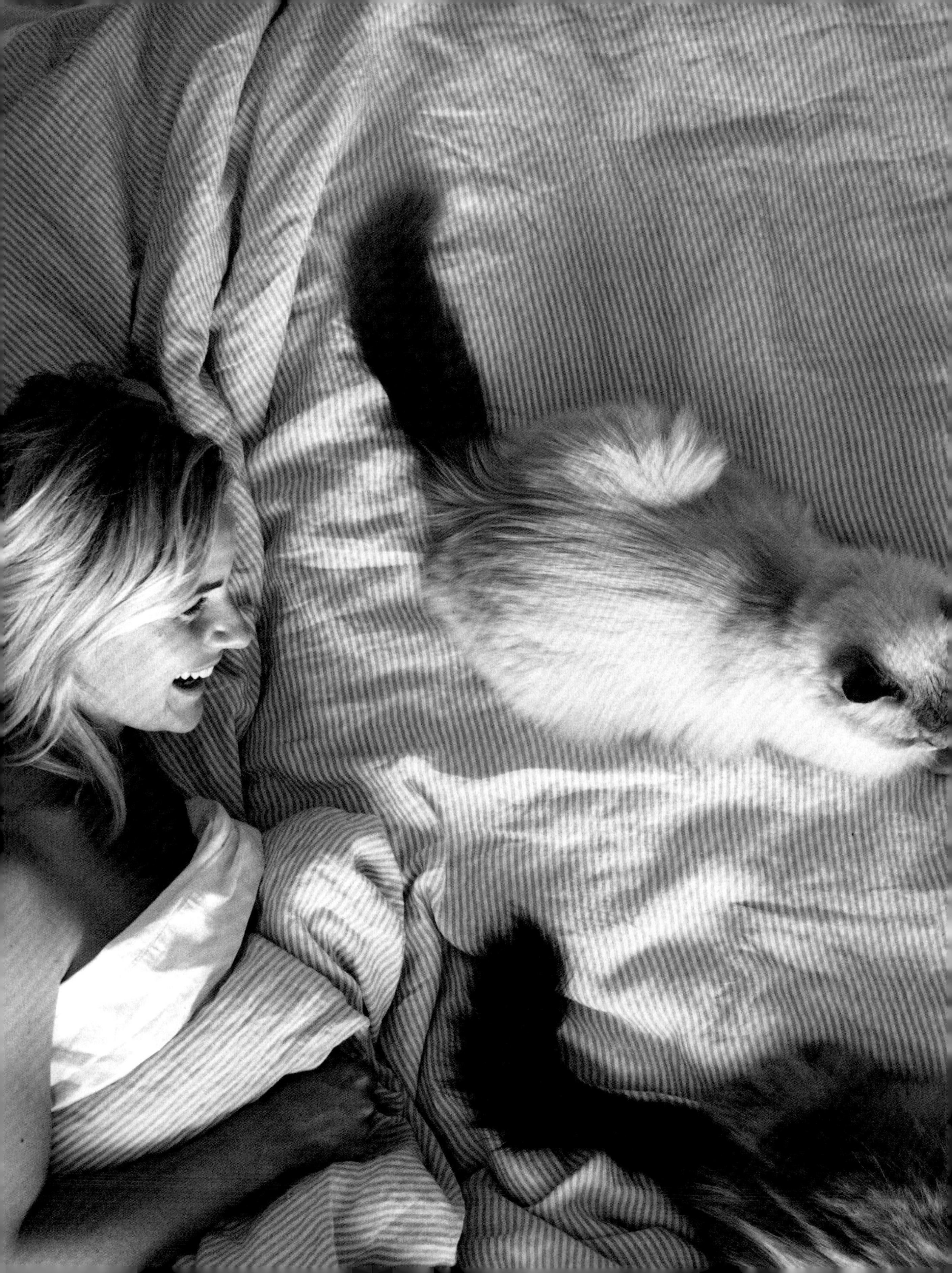

the effect that one night of lost sleep had on anxiety and emotion regulation in eighteen healthy young adults. The study participants who were totally deprived of one night of sleep reported a 30 per cent increase in anxiety levels, while those who had a full night's sleep reported no rise whatsoever. This difference was also picked up in the participants' brain scans, which showed that the sleep-deprived individuals had more activity in their amygdalae—the brain centre of fear and anxiety.

Additionally, in response to watching a video clip that was supposed to bring about emotion, the sleep-deprived participants also had much *less* activity in the area of their brain that is responsible for regulating emotions. This suggested that sleep may help us to keep a hold on our emotions. So, if you've ever felt like a right emotional mess after a night of no sleep, this may well explain why.

SLEEP HYGIENE

You might have heard the term 'sleep hygiene' before, and if you haven't it's pretty simple. It's essentially a collection of tips and tricks that can help you to form healthy habits around sleep, in order to get yourself the best night's sleep humanly possible.

Art and I have employed some of these tricks in our household—and I'll tell you what, I thought I was a good sleeper before, but even I've improved with the help of some of these!

*   Try to get into a routine of going to bed at the same time each night and waking up at the same time each morning. (Maybe excluding weekends or Sundays, because who doesn't need a good sleep-in every now and again?) Sticking to a set bedtime and wake-up time helps your body's circadian rhythm get sussed.

✳ Establish a relaxing bedtime routine. A regular routine right before you go to bed lets your body know that it's sleepy time. This might take the form of a warm shower or bath every night before getting into bed, or reading a book and/or stretching.

✳ Avoid naps during the day, if you can. (Again, this one may be easier if you're sans young children!) Naps can mess with that circadian rhythm of yours.

✳ Don't have a TV in your room. As tempting as it might be, having a TV in your room isn't a great idea. Try to keep your bedroom a calm place of sleep—not too hot or cold, and not a lot of light or loud noise. These things can all disrupt a restful sleep.

✳ If you're feeling smug because you don't even have a TV, this applies to laptops too! I know Netflix in bed might sound like a fabulous idea, but it's not going to help you get to sleep. Quite the opposite, in fact. If you have trouble saying no to the next episode (and the next, and the next), then you should probably keep your binge-watching habits to the living room.

✳ Do some form of exercise every day. I know I've already mentioned how incredible exercise is for your health and well-being, but it honestly can do wonders for your sleep by getting you good and tired and ready for bed at the end of the day.

✳ Avoid caffeine later in the day. A lot of people will say that an afternoon coffee is fine because they don't get much of a buzz from caffeine—but, if this is you, and you're having trouble getting a decent sleep every night, then maybe it's time to try removing the caffeine from your afternoons. See if it helps.

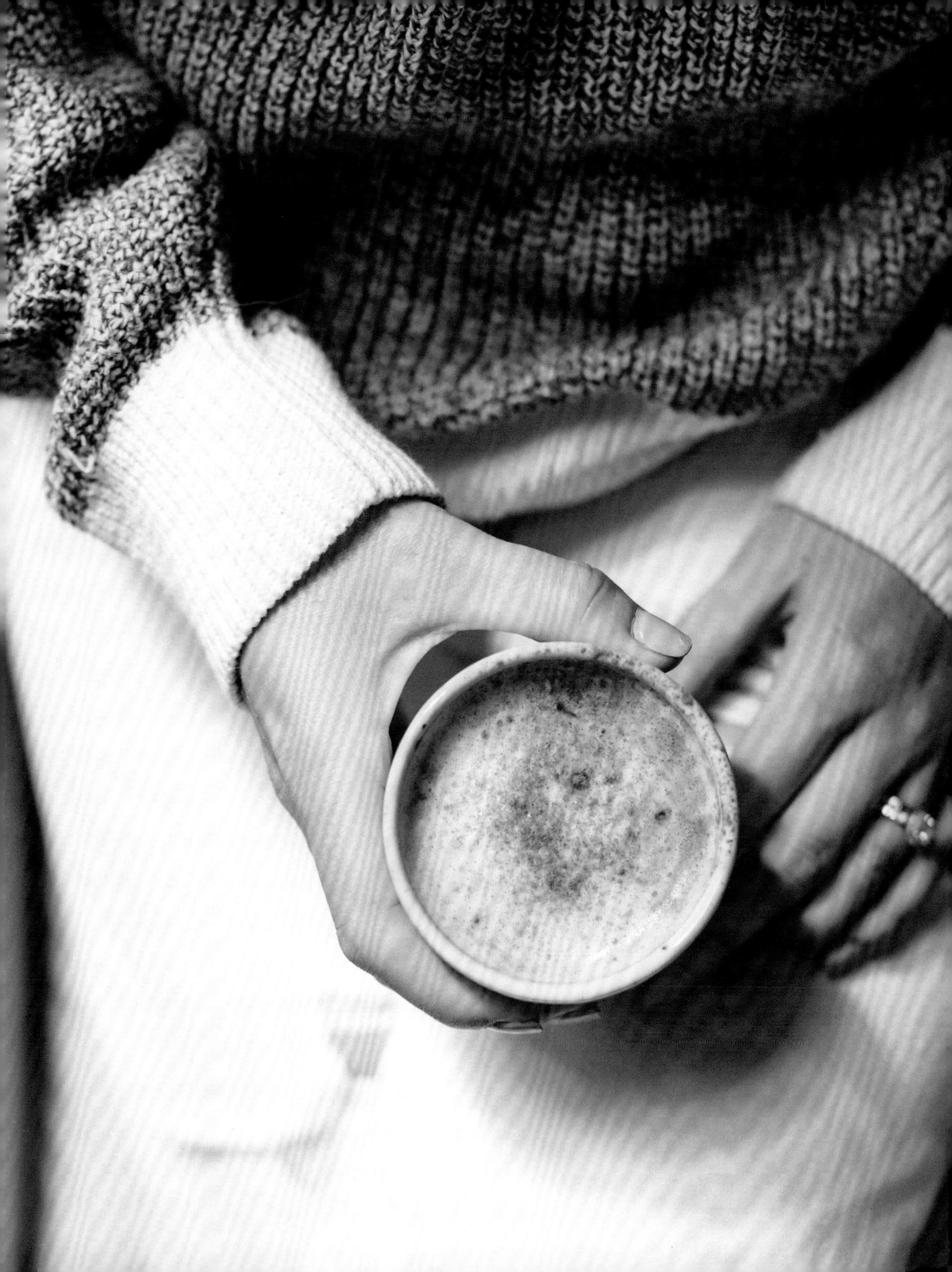

Screen time is just one of many
fantastic parts of modern life,
but we need to learn how to
get a bit of balance with it.

NO PHONES AT BEDTIME

A major barrier to a good sleep these days is—you guessed it—screen time. There's a heap of evidence for this. For instance, a study published in the peer-reviewed medical journal *Acta Paediatrica* looked at the association between social media and sleep duration among a group of Canadian students aged between eleven and 20. The researchers concluded that greater use of social media was associated with shorter sleep duration.

Part of the reason that spending time staring at a screen can negatively impact your sleep is because of the blue light that screens give off. This light, especially when combined with the stimulating content that your social media feeds serve up in an attempt to keep you scrolling, can make it really hard for your body to slow down and relax for sleepy time.

'What the heck is blue light?' I hear you ask. Well, remember how I said earlier that artificial light can mess with your circadian rhythm? That's complicated by the fact that not all light colours (or wavelengths) are created equal. Light sources that emit blue light include the sun, electronics such as your phone or computer, and LED and fluorescent lighting. Blue light is helpful during the daytime, because it can boost your attention, reaction times and mood, but those benefits quickly turn to problems when you're trying to get some sleep at night-time. Of course, electronics with screens are EVERYWHERE, and so is energy-efficient lighting, so we're exposed to blue wavelengths after sundown now more than ever.

It's well established that light of any kind suppresses your body's secretion of melatonin, but blue light at night does so even more powerfully than other wavelengths. Melatonin is a hormone that, among other things, helps to control your body's circadian rhythm. One experiment conducted by Harvard researchers found that exposure to blue light suppressed melatonin for about twice as long as exposure to green light did. What's more, exposure to blue light also shifted circadian rhythms by twice as much.

What all this suggests is that it's probably better to stay away from screens right before bed. Screen time is just one of many fantastic parts of modern life, but we need to learn how to get a bit of balance with it. If it's impacting the basic things we need as humans—quality sleep being a major one—then the way we use it probably needs to be adjusted.

As we've discussed, quality sleep plays a major role in pretty much every aspect of our lives. Do we really want to let scrolling through our phones impact that? I think we know which of those things should be our priority, right?

For some tips to help you get a good night's sleep, see my sleep action plan on the next page.

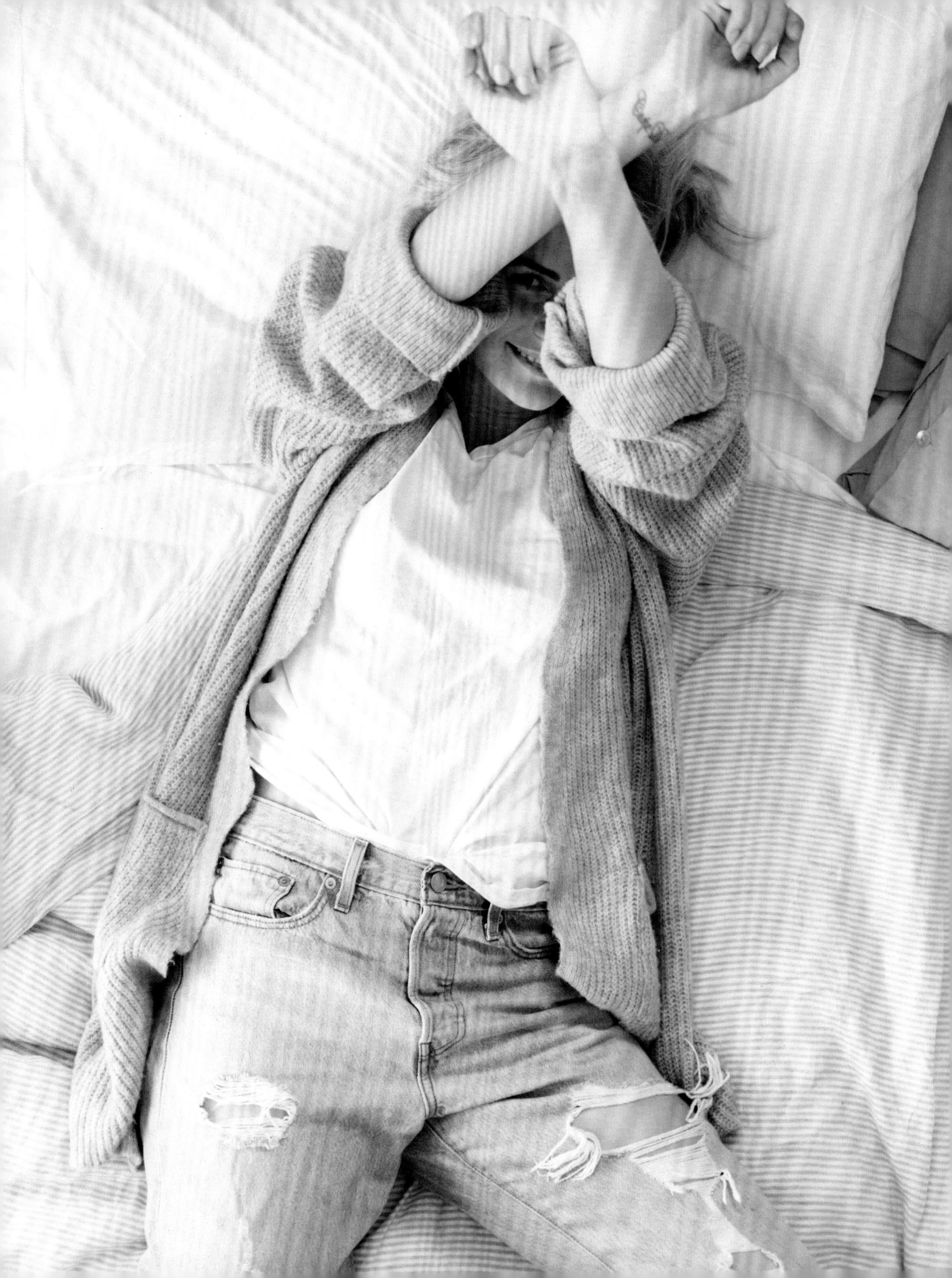

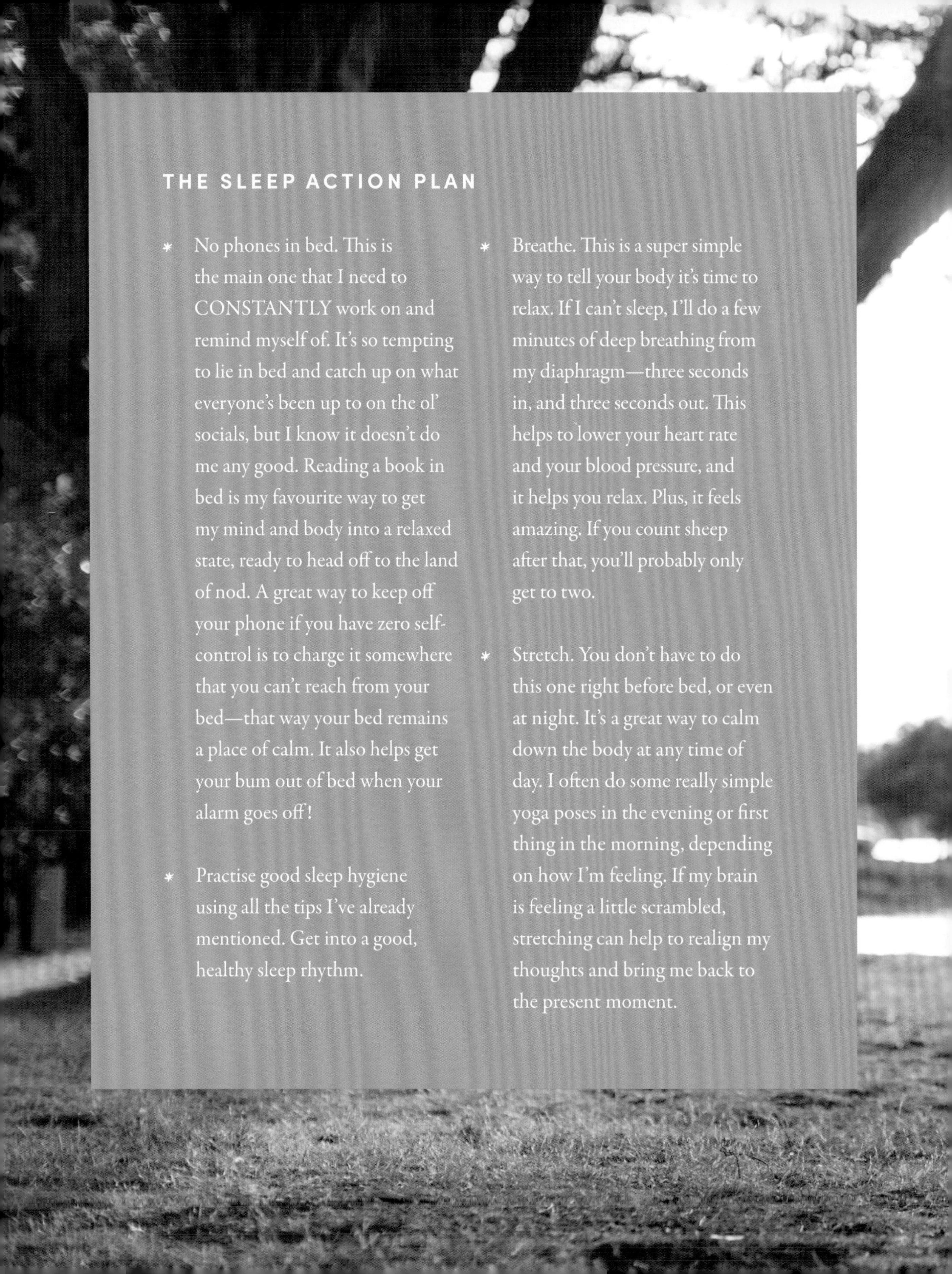

THE SLEEP ACTION PLAN

* No phones in bed. This is the main one that I need to CONSTANTLY work on and remind myself of. It's so tempting to lie in bed and catch up on what everyone's been up to on the ol' socials, but I know it doesn't do me any good. Reading a book in bed is my favourite way to get my mind and body into a relaxed state, ready to head off to the land of nod. A great way to keep off your phone if you have zero self-control is to charge it somewhere that you can't reach from your bed—that way your bed remains a place of calm. It also helps get your bum out of bed when your alarm goes off!

* Practise good sleep hygiene using all the tips I've already mentioned. Get into a good, healthy sleep rhythm.

* Breathe. This is a super simple way to tell your body it's time to relax. If I can't sleep, I'll do a few minutes of deep breathing from my diaphragm—three seconds in, and three seconds out. This helps to lower your heart rate and your blood pressure, and it helps you relax. Plus, it feels amazing. If you count sheep after that, you'll probably only get to two.

* Stretch. You don't have to do this one right before bed, or even at night. It's a great way to calm down the body at any time of day. I often do some really simple yoga poses in the evening or first thing in the morning, depending on how I'm feeling. If my brain is feeling a little scrambled, stretching can help to realign my thoughts and bring me back to the present moment.

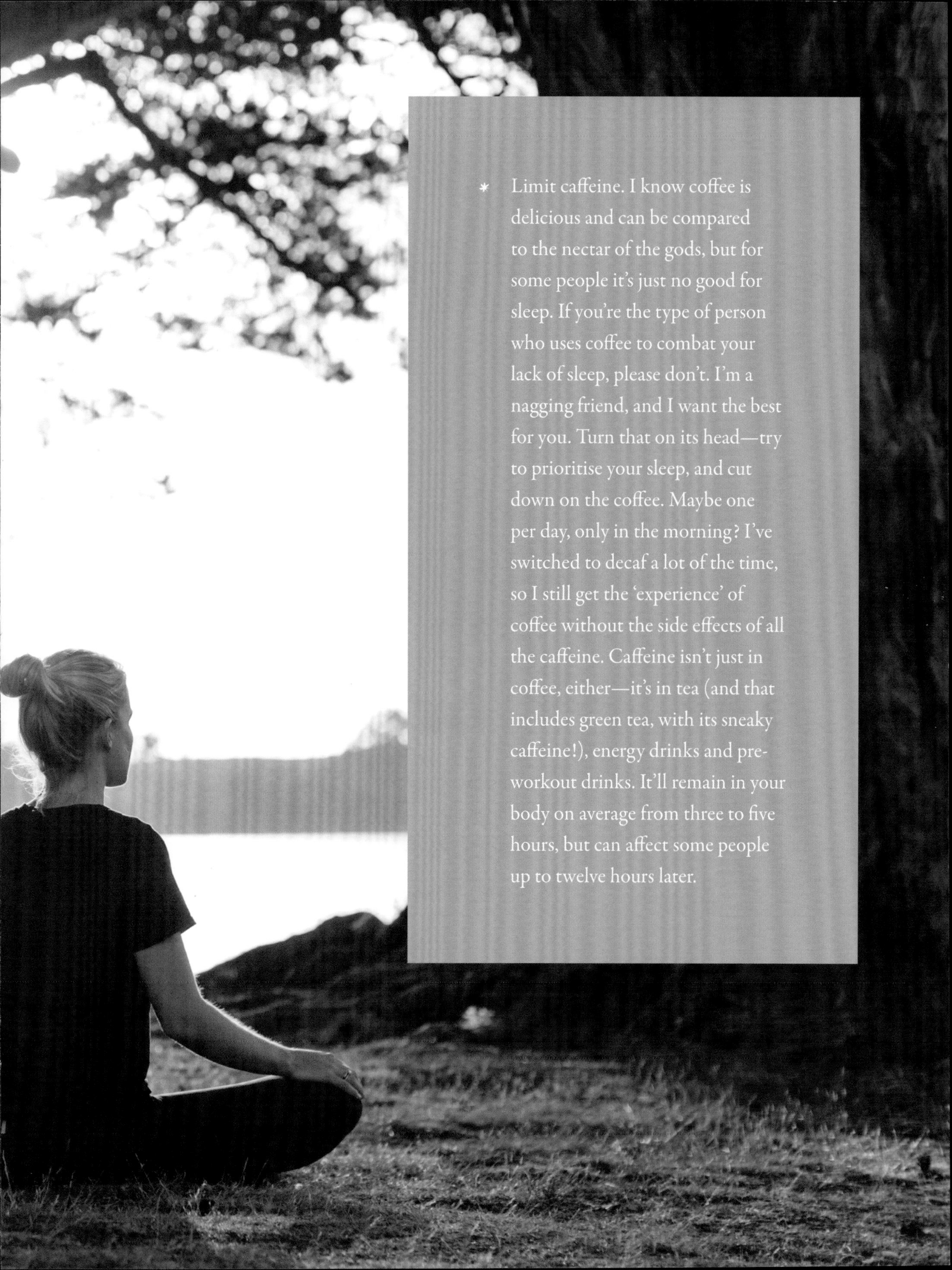

* Limit caffeine. I know coffee is delicious and can be compared to the nectar of the gods, but for some people it's just no good for sleep. If you're the type of person who uses coffee to combat your lack of sleep, please don't. I'm a nagging friend, and I want the best for you. Turn that on its head—try to prioritise your sleep, and cut down on the coffee. Maybe one per day, only in the morning? I've switched to decaf a lot of the time, so I still get the 'experience' of coffee without the side effects of all the caffeine. Caffeine isn't just in coffee, either—it's in tea (and that includes green tea, with its sneaky caffeine!), energy drinks and pre-workout drinks. It'll remain in your body on average from three to five hours, but can affect some people up to twelve hours later.

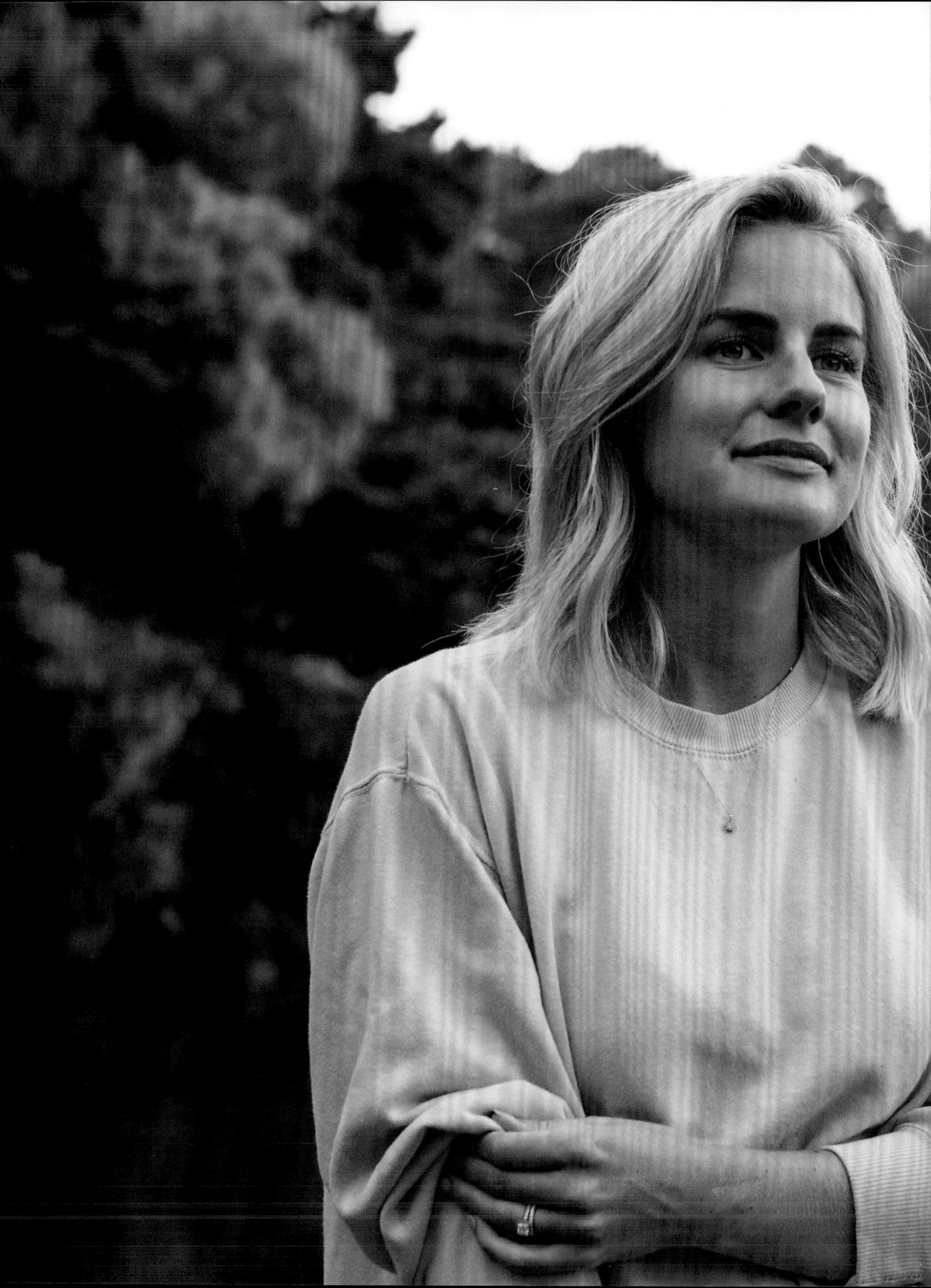

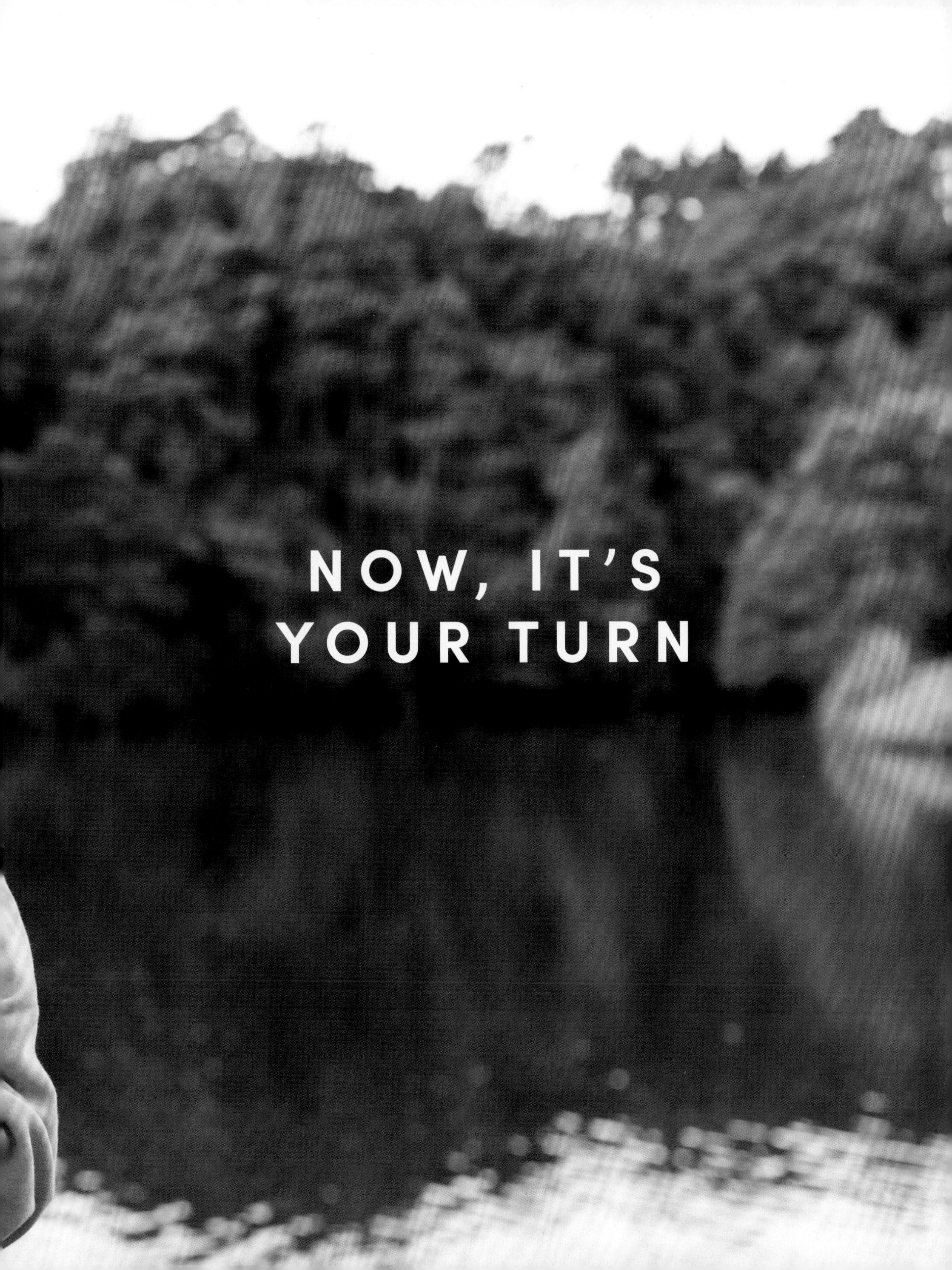

NOW, IT'S YOUR TURN

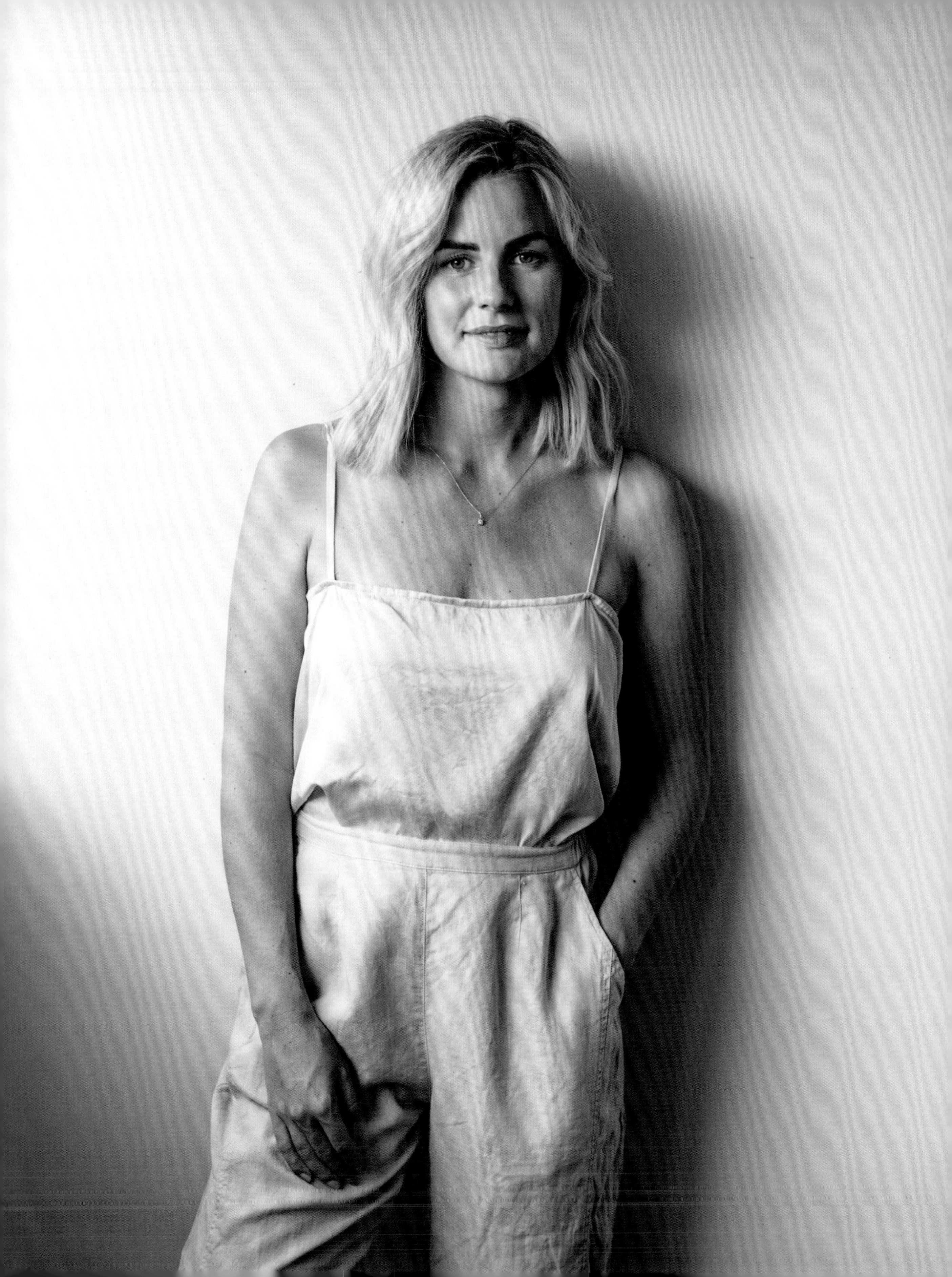

You've officially reached the end of the book! By now, you've learnt all about how your happiness and your self-esteem are connected, and you've read about the things I've done (and still do) to keep my self-esteem and well-being on point in this crazy, social-media-saturated world.

That means it's your turn! I hope you feel like your personal toolbox has been filled with all the knowledge and practical action points that you need to build the strongest self-esteem you've ever had. I hope you feel prepared to go out into the world, your confidence in your pocket, and tackle the big and small challenges that life throws at you. I hope you've got a refreshed, optimistic and hopeful outlook on life, and a super-positive sense of self.

I tell you what, it's not an easy task admitting that your self-esteem may need a bit of work. I bloody salute you for having the self-awareness to see it, and the motivation to do something about it. That takes guts, and it's awesome that you're keen to learn with me.

When I started writing this book, I thought I had a lot to share—but, the more I wrote, the more I realised I still had work to do myself. I saw that I still had areas where I could make changes and improvements. As a result, I really feel like this book has been a shared journey. You and me, we've been through it together. I'm so excited for us to feel awesome about ourselves together.

Personal development is not always easy or straightforward. It's not something that happens overnight. It's a constant work in progress. We are never going to be perfect, because perfect doesn't exist. And, anyway, who'd want to be perfect? Where would the fun be in that? We can, however, always try to improve how we feel about ourselves. Personal growth is a fantastic thing. So long as we're all trying and doing a little bit better than we were yesterday, then that sounds pretty good to me.

Feeling good about yourself can literally change your life, and the one person who is in control of your self-esteem is *you*. I hope you know how beautiful you really are, and how much you have to offer this world. As soon as you believe that truth, the world will become your oyster. You'll have the courage to go after the things you truly want in life, and the determination to grab the life that you desire—which is the life that you deserve—with both hands.

So what are you waiting for?

Go get it!

Feeling good about yourself can literally change your life, and the one person who is in control of your self-esteem is *you*. I hope you know how beautiful you really are, and how much you have to offer this world.

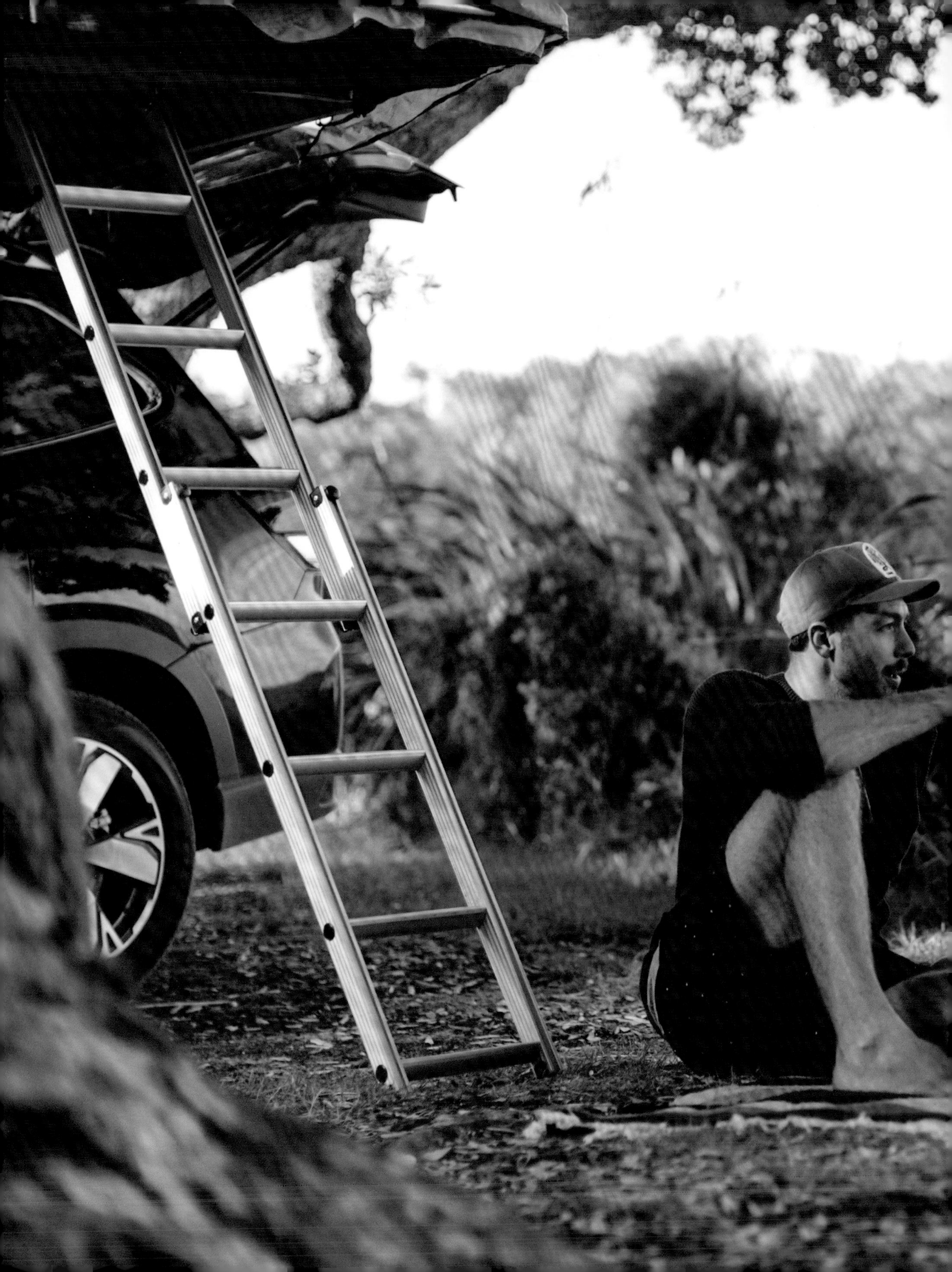

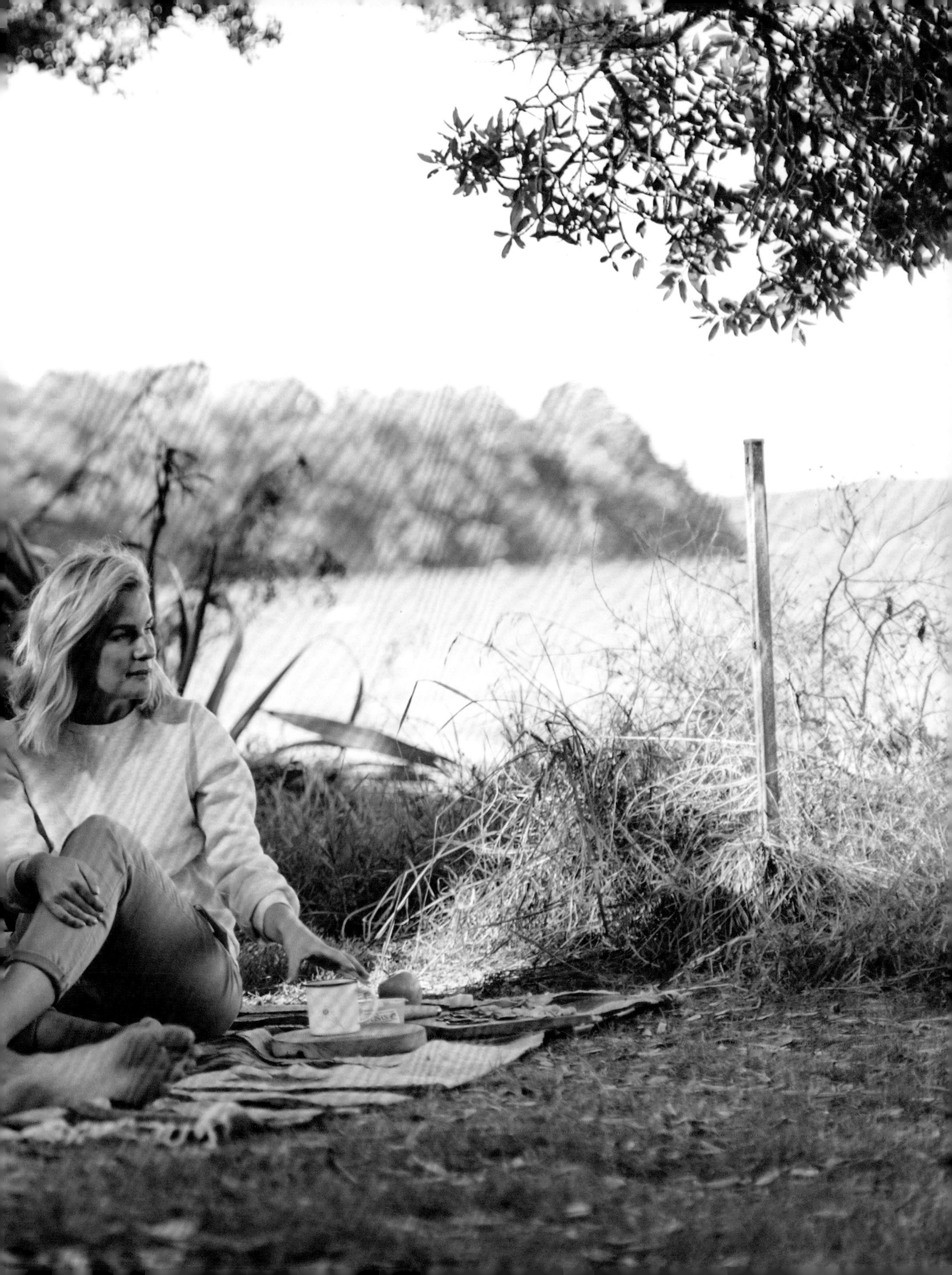

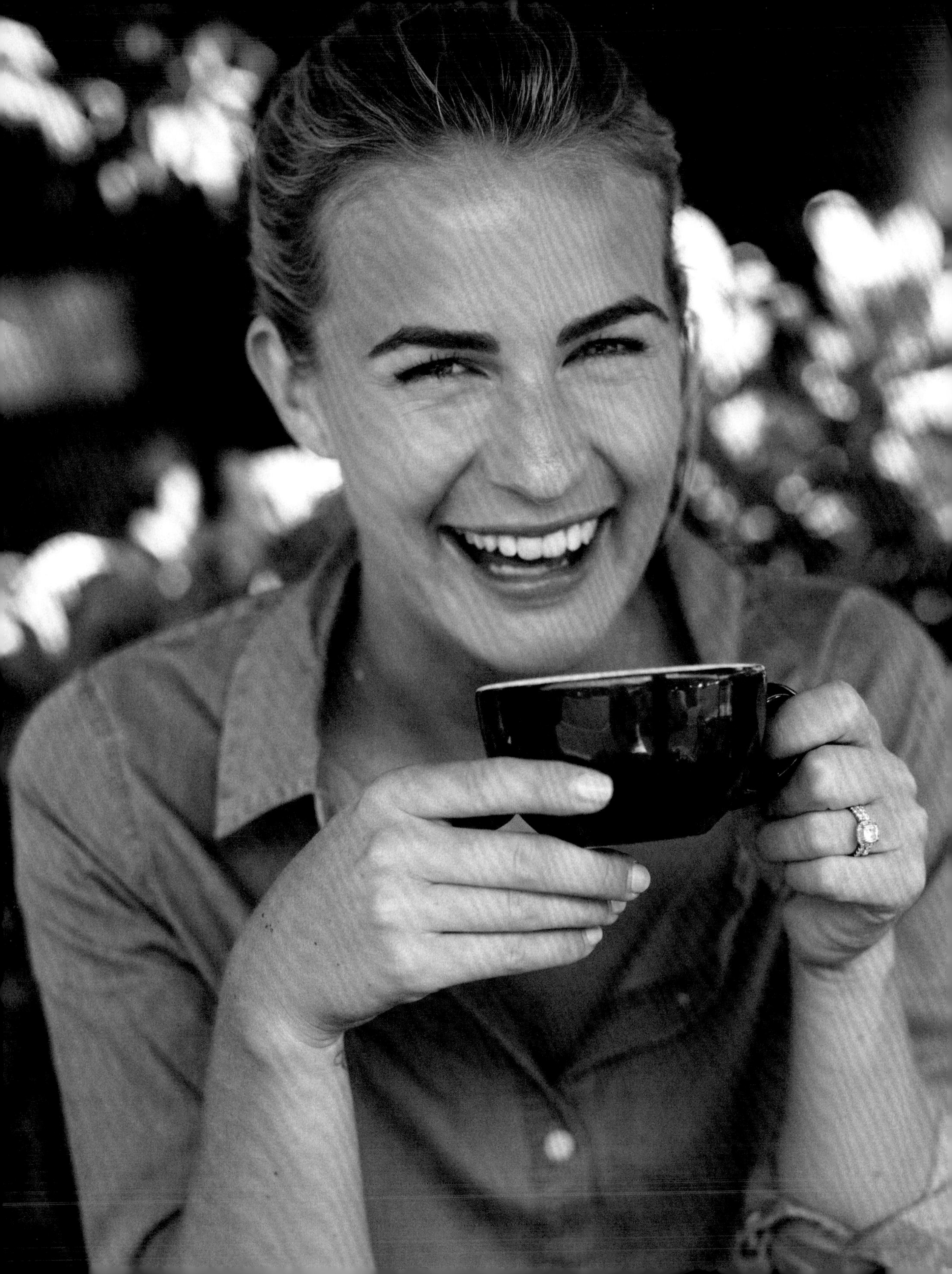

ACKNOWLEDGEMENTS

First off, I just want to say how proud I am of this book! I really hope you loved reading it as much as I loved writing it. In the process of writing this book, however, one thing I did discover is that it's remarkably difficult to focus for long periods of time while pregnant . . . But, hey, we got there.

This book simply wouldn't be what it is without the remarkable Kimberley Davis, my editor. Thank you so much for all your ideas and encouragement. I think we make quite a good team!

Thank you also to Jenny Hellen, and the team at Allen & Unwin. You guys are so lovely to work with, and I feel very lucky that I've been able to publish not one but TWO books with you. All because you had faith in me.

Thank you to Emily Hlaváč Green for all the stunning photography, and for helping me with creative direction. You are one bloody talented lady, and the best sister-in-law I could ask for. Thank you also to Kate Barraclough for designing the pages so beautifully, and for bringing my vision of the book to life.

And last, but certainly not least, to my husband, Art. Thank you for your constant support. On the days when I doubted myself, you always had the perfect words of encouragement. Quite the skill, I believe. Our son is incredibly lucky to have you as a dad.

Oh, one more actually – thank you to YOU, the lovely reader, for buying (or borrowing) this book. I really do appreciate your support.

x

SOME FEEL-GOOD RESOURCES

Websites

greatergood.berkeley.edu *Greater Good Magazine* is published by the Greater Good Science Center at the University of California, Berkeley. The magazine (to use their own words), 'turns scientific research into stories, tips, and tools for a happier life and a more compassionate society'. The website is chocka with articles covering a wide range of topics.

drhyman.com The personal website of Dr Mark Hyman, the director at Cleveland Clinic's Center for Functional Medicine and Founder of The UltraWellness Center. He's incredibly knowledgeable on all things nutrition, and on wellness in general. He is one of my go-to gurus. He also has a really interesting podcast called *The Doctor's Farmacy*.

doyouyoga.com I love yoga, but sometimes I just can't be bothered getting out of my pyjamas and going to a class. This is an awesome website with lots of online classes that you can do at home. You can either do it straight off your laptop or phone, or cast it to your telly.

sleepfoundation.org The website of the US National Sleep Foundation contains a bunch of useful information about—yep, you guessed it—sleep, including suggestions for getting a good night's rest.

resource-project.org The website for The ReSource Project, a unique large-scale study on Eastern and Western methods of mental training.

Apps

headspace.com
calm.com
1giantmind.com
themindfulnessapp.com
mindworks.org
insighttimer.com
For more info on all of these apps, see pages 96–98.

My favourite travel accounts

@beautifuldestinations If you love some good old-fashioned Earth porn, you will love this account. They travel all over the world taking stunning photos that will put you in awe of our planet!

@natgeo and @natgeotravel These two *National Geographic* accounts are really great, with interesting captions that give you some 'behind the lens' insight.

@travellingthroughtheworld An account filled with magical travel photos that always makes me feel something special!

@kylefinndempsey I've followed this guy for years. He posts awesome photos, and we've actually got a couple of his photos up as prints at home. I find a lot of travel bloggers take similar photos with a similar edit, but this guy does his own thing and his photos feel a bit more personal.

@carmenhuter I had the pleasure of meeting Carmen earlier this year, and both her passion for the planet and her INSANE photography skills are really inspiring.

@lola.photography Another friend of mine, Lola's photos of mainly New Zealand landscapes are so dreamy and colourful.

My favourite positivity accounts
@the_happy_broadcast A really awesome page presenting positive things that are happening all over the world, but which we may not hear about in the media.

@happsters A lovely lady named Kelli who posts about beautiful, positive things going on in the world.

@humansofny You might have heard of this account, as it went viral years ago on Facebook and became a book. It posts real-world photos and stories of the different types of people living in New York City.

@happynotperfect These guys also have a mindfulness app, but I love their Instagram. It's filled with lovely quotes, and just general life inspo.

My favourite mindfulness accounts
@deepakchopra Deepk Chopra has been around a long time, and is a huge advocate of the mind–body connection. He's pretty far along on his spirituality journey, though, so I have to think about some of his posts for a good 24 hours to even slightly understand them . . . but I love them all the same.

@lightworkerslounge This is the Instagram page for the podcast of the same name, and I love the light-hearted way they post about spirituality. They get a great message across, and do it in a fun, approachable way.

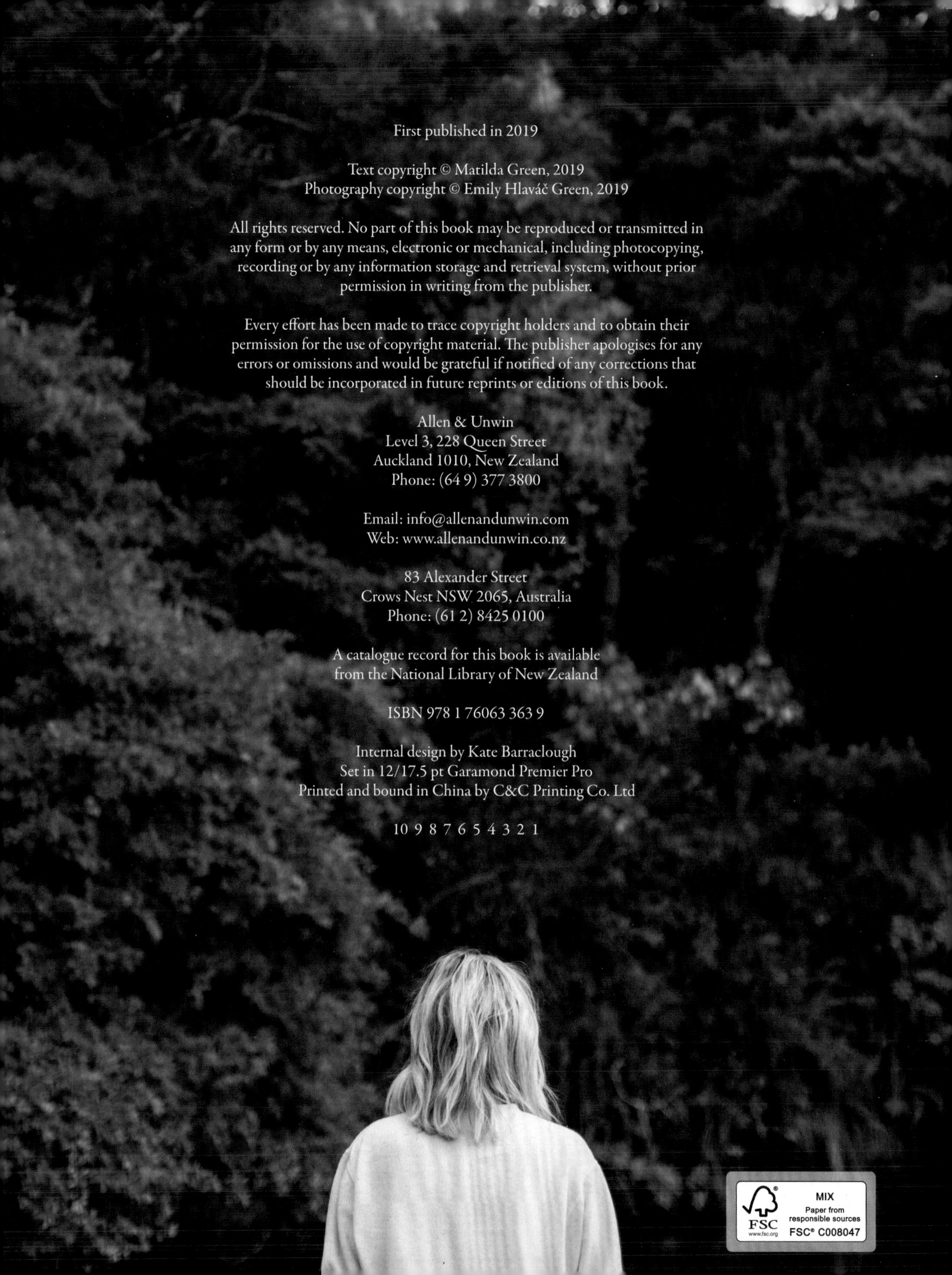

First published in 2019

Allen & Unwin
Level 3, 228 Queen Street
Auckland 1010, New Zealand
Phone: (64 9) 377 3800

Email: info@allenandunwin.com
Web: www.allenandunwin.co.nz

83 Alexander Street
Crows Nest NSW 2065, Australia
Phone: (61 2) 8425 0100

A catalogue record for this book is available
from the National Library of New Zealand

ISBN 978 1 76063 363 9

Internal design by Kate Barraclough
Set in 12/17.5 pt Garamond Premier Pro
Printed and bound in China by C&C Printing Co. Ltd

10 9 8 7 6 5 4 3 2 1

MIX
Paper from
responsible sources
FSC® C008047